The Bariatric Foodie
Holiday Survival Guide

Ordering Information:
Quantity sales. Special discounts are available on quantity purchases by corporations, associations and others. Book signings and appearances can be arranged directly by the author by contacting (443) 486-2301 or bariatricfoodie@yahoo.com.

www.BariatricFoodie.com

Printed in the United States of America.

The Bariatric Foodie Holiday Survival Guide.

ISBN: 978-0-9910770-0-7

Table of Contents

Acknowledgments

No Bariatric Foodie™ book would ever get published were it not for the generosity of many, many, many people. That is to say, even if you are not listed here, I appreciate your help and value your friendship!

To Pamela Tremble, award-winning graphic designer, thank you for another great book cover. You have been the driving force behind Bariatric Foodie's visual look, brand and a large contributor to its success.

To Kelly Morris, a most conscientious copy editor. I don't make her work easy, but I do very much appreciate her insight and attention to detail. Thank you!

To Julia Weaver, who laid out this book. Thank you! I don't think I could have possible worked with this text another minute! You saved me.

And last, but most certainly not least, to Joy Muller, who made sure that my inclusion of kosher-appropriate recipes in this book was also culturally appropriate. I am so thankful you are a part of the Foodie Nation!

It's the Holidays!
(Don't freak out!)

It's the holidays. And you've had weight loss surgery.

And up until this point you've been very positive about all the changes you've gone through. You've been eating your protein first. Sipping water to try and reach your water goals. Taking your vitamins and moving your butt.

But all that sort of seems like a moot point when you come face to face with Aunt So-and-So's famous Yule Log. Or your mom's famous sweet potato casserole made with maple syrup. Or any of the myriad holiday foods that will either make you violently ill or wreck your weight loss progress.

I feel your pain. I've been there.

Picture it. Maryland. November 2008. Nikki was 10 months post-op. While my eating capacity had improved since surgery in January, I still couldn't eat enough to "pass for normal," especially not at an African-American Thanksgiving celebration!

But thankfully the universe was on my side. My stepsister Crystal decided to come up from North Carolina for the holiday. Why is that significant? Well, that year she was a cast member on Survivor: Gabon. So needless to say her presence made me nearly invisible, something that in a past life I might resent but for which, in this particular year, I was profoundly thankful!

For you (unless you have relatives on reality TV), the holidays are likely to draw scrutiny about how much and what you can eat. So what do you do?

You make a plan! And I'm here to help.

But wait. I'm getting ahead of myself. Many of you probably don't even know who I am. My name is Nikki and, like I said, I had gastric bypass surgery in January 2008. I'm maintaining a 130 lbs. weight loss (yay me!). I also run a site called Bariatric Foodie that helps other weight loss surgery patients learn to "play with their food."

What the heck do I mean by that? I mean that most dishes we love can be recreated in healthier ways. We just have to put some thought into exactly what we like about the dish and be open minded enough to translate that into different forms. I know what you're thinking right now. "Yeah. Right."

Another true story. Picture it. Maryland. 2012. Family Christmas Potluck. My contribution? A pan of my four-cheese mashed cauliflower (recipe included!). I had one particularly vocal family member who proclaimed he KNEW he'd hate the side dish. Then he tasted a little bit of it and...well...let's just say I lost count of how many times he went up for another helping and he quietly exited the dinner early, taking my pan of cheesy cauliflower goodness with him!

So it can be done. And I'm going to show you how. But I'm also going to break down the dynamics of the holidays and what can make them so stressful to you, the person trying to lose weight. We'll go over social dynamics, the politics of recipes and more —all very fascinating stuff!

All this is to say that I know many people have specific dishes that are traditional to your family or your culture or your geographic region. I can't begin to cover every holiday dish known to man. But what I can give you is ideas on how you can change your dishes for the better and how to cope when everything seems to revolve around food!

You up for the challenge? If so, turn the page and let's get started!

Section One:
The Holiday Head Game

Why Your Efforts at Healthier Holiday Cooking *Will* Be Met With Resistance (And what to do about it)

In my four years of experience as a blogger and nearly six years of experience as a post-op bariatric patient, I've learned that families can have a variety of reactions to the proposition of healthier eating.

- They can embrace it wholeheartedly.
- They can reject it outright.
- They can go into it tentatively, but adventurously.

And the tricky thing is that they can employ any of these three attitudes at various points. One day they may love your healthier dishes, the next day they may reject them outright.

But all this seems to change around the holidays. Around the holidays, it seems, most proposals to change recipes (especially iconic ones) are met with fierce resistance!

What's an iconic recipe?

Generally speaking, an iconic recipe is one that lives in your mind, memory and taste buds in a very specific way. It may be your mom's perfectly roasted turkey. Your aunt's famous stuffing. So far as general audiences, green bean casserole is a good example. When we say green bean casserole, many Americans conjure up a specific image: a casserole dish filled with verdant green beans mixed with cream soup and topped with French-fried onions and cheese. Am I right?

It's when we mess with those kinds of recipes that people tend to get testy.

Why do people react the way they do to changing iconic recipes?

The thing we often forget (or maybe even shun) after weight loss surgery is the fact that food is more than just food. It's more than just fuel for our bodies. In the foods we eat, there are years — maybe even centuries and millennia — of history, culture and tradition.

And that's okay. No…really it is!

That being the case, people take iconic recipes very seriously. They treasure the recipes because in making those recipes they are participating in a ritual that connects them to people who lived before them and people who will live after them. It's a sacred thing. And we tend to be protective of sacred things.

What does this mean to you?

- It means that you should be thoughtful about how you change a recipe to make it healthier — or even whether you advertise that it is healthier. The next section will go into more detail.
- It also means that you have to be patient with your family. Sometimes taste and memory are inextricably linked and in their minds, simply because it isn't the same recipe they've always had, it just doesn't taste as good. Try to be understanding and don't take it personally!
- Know and accept that there are some recipes that are just sacred (for many reasons) and that you should not touch them! You can either make a smaller batch of a modified recipe for yourself or you can have a small amount of the real thing.

Now all this is a moot point if you have a family of culinary adventurers. If you do, I envy you! Getting my own family to accept some healthier variations of recipes has been rough at times. But it's well worth the effort.

Just remember, the holidays are about family, tradition and love. Keep those three things at the heart of what you do and you really can't go wrong!

The Art of Covert Cooking

It sounds illicit, doesn't it? Covert cooking. And it kind of is!

When I say covert cooking, I mean that your mission, should you choose to accept it, is to produce a dish that looks, smells, tastes and feels like the original recipe, but with better ingredients! There are several guiding principles to covert cooking that you should be aware of before you decide if this route is right for you.

- I said this before but the point bears repeating, the dish should appear the same as the original!
- This means that you have to be smart about swapping and that the final product, while healthier, may not pass rigid post-op standards. But this is the holidays, so that's okay!
- By nature, covert cooking is done in secret. You generally don't tell people you covert cooked something. Or at least not while they are eating it. It's hard to stay quiet but you can ruin your outcome by spilling the beans too soon!

With that knowledge in hand let's discuss how you approach this endeavor. Most of us know our holiday recipes like the back of our hands. We've made them for years and we could probably make them in our sleep. Still step one is write down your recipe. This practice can bring to light some very obvious changes you can make right away.

In my estimation, the easiest swaps to make are:

- A lean meat for a fattier one (if the moisture of the dish is affected by the use of ultra-lean meat, replace ¾ of the meat with lean and leave ¼ regular).
- Greek yogurt as a substitute for sour cream.
- Reduced fat (not fat free!) cheese for full-fat cheese.
- Reduced fat milk or cream (not fat free!) for full-fat milk or cream.
- Reduced fat soups and broths.

Conversely the swaps that don't go over so well are:

- Trying to completely remove the starch. (Don't try to pass off cheesy mashed cauliflower as mac 'n cheese. It just never works!)
- Trying to replace something that was high fat with something that is completely fat free (fat has flavor and moisture).
- Blindly adding protein powder to things (there is protein powder in some of the recipes I've outlined but very specific instructions on how to add it!).
- Replacing all the sugar in a recipe with sugar substitute. Unless your family is accustomed to the taste of a sugar substitute, they are going to notice!

So how do you get around those challenges and still make a dish you feel good about?

- Instead of replacing the starch, try using a better starch. Use a high-fiber or whole grain starch in your dishes wherever possible. For rice, use brown instead of white. For potatoes, try using red-skinned, which offer some additional nutrients.
- For fat content, as I said with the meat, you can usually get away with replacing most of the fatty product in a recipe with reduced fat. Sometimes for flavor and texture you need to use some of the full fat product. The recipes in this book will note when that is the case.
- Unless you've tested a recipe that incorporates protein powder, don't do it. It's too risky!
- Instead of replacing a lot of sugar, I'd suggest cutting back on sugar. You can even use a blend of sugar substitute and real sugar (Splenda sells such a product and so does Wal-Mart in its Great Value brand). You can also use honey or Stevia. This doesn't really lower your carb count but at least you know what's in your food. You can also play off the sweetness of the fruits you use in recipes to achieve sweetness.

There is also a sub-set of covert cooking whereby you make your dishes in the traditional way and then a smaller portion in the healthier way (and in this case you can go nuts with the healthy recipe) and advertise that the recipe is "just for you." Somehow the "it's not mine" mentality takes over and people want to try it and like it.

This can cause a problem for you if you've not gotten a portion but it's a good way to get the family to at least take a taste of the healthier version. Anyone who reads Bariatric Foodie knows this sub-set of covert cooking is why my Apple Brown Nik (page 87) is such a hit during the holidays now!

Like I said before, you don't have to covert cook. You can either just make a dish healthier, let your family know and challenge them to deal with it or you are always welcome to make your traditional dishes the way you've always done. The holidays are all about moderation. As long as you aren't eating this stuff year round, there is absolutely nothing wrong with a special treat! But it is that, a treat. And an occasional one.

Surviving the Holidays with Your Sanity Intact

We all know that food is about more than being hungry, don't we? (Please say yes!)

In part, we know this because, for those of us who experience extreme restriction after weight loss surgery, eating is decidedly un-fun. It's often marked by feelings of deprivation (you didn't eat enough to satisfy your brain), apathy (why should I cook something special when I can only take three bites?) and fear (dumping syndrome, at least in the beginning, can make eating feel like a game of Russian roulette).

Then, there's your family to deal with. As I said earlier, we're dealing with iconic recipes that they are attached to. You'll have to deal with that. But you'll also likely deal with a fair amount of scrutiny, whether you've shared about your surgery or not, because you've changed, probably a lot, since the last time any of these people last saw you!

Don't get overwhelmed. It's possible to get through the holidays without losing your mind! Let's talk about this, starting with the mother of all American glutton holidays.

Thanksgiving

Oh, Turkey Day! Thanksgiving is a holiday for counting our blessings, enjoying our family and, traditionally, sharing an outrageously large and over-caloric meal. It's the American way and no amount of self-help talk can get us around that.

But if you are a Bariatric Foodie you know you should always, always have a strategy.

To that effect here are some tips to get you up to, and through, Thanksgiving without going crazy, falling completely off the wagon or depriving yourself of the wonderful foods the holiday has to offer.

Turkey Day Tip #1: "He (or She) who makes the meal, determines the meal content."

...but that does NOT mean you have to go around advertising your first annual healthy Thanksgiving dinner. We know you are excited about all the wonderful and healthy recipes and cooking methods you've learned (and we hope you learned a good deal of them here), but the fastest way to turn a non-op off is to advertise that something is healthy. For whatever reason, it translates in their minds as bland and flavorless. While you don't have to covert cook, as prescribed in the last section, you might not want to use a bullhorn to announce your first healthy Thanksgiving.

Here's the key to making that work without (technically) lying. Put the food on the table (or buffet...or counter...or whatever you use to serve) and then walk away! Say nothing. Let people enjoy the food. We always feel we need to "warn" people that something is healthy, but why? Unless there is a real reason to let someone know (say, they are allergic to sugar substitutes), what they don't know won't hurt them.

Turkey Day Tip #2: At the family dinner, learn the "Rules of Three's."

What are the rules of three's? There are two from our perspective (thought we were gonna say there were three rules, didn't you?): The "three bite rule" and the "three minute" rule.

The "three bite rule"-This is geared toward moderation. When facing a room full of food you think you can't have, one of three things is bound to happen. Either you will a) get really moody because you feel resentful b) your obvious longing for the food will make everyone else uncomfortable eating it or c) you'll set yourself up to think you are "cheating" which usually results in over-indulgence. Instead, re-write that story! You can have whatever you want from the dinner table. Eat a bit of protein first and then with the more carby stuff, allow yourself approximately three bites of it. Want some pumpkin pie? Three bites. Want that homemade mac 'n cheese? Three bites!

Newbies: if you don't know what you dump on yet (or even if you dump) go straight to the next rule.

The "three minute rule"-This rule can be a pain in the butt. But it's saved me from getting sick so many times I can't even tell you. If there is something served where you don't know if you will dump, take a bite. Chew it, swallow it. Then wait three minutes. That's long enough to let your pouch (or sleeve, or stomach or whatever you call your anatomy) have its reaction. If nothing happens, proceed with caution. Eat slowly and chew well. If you feel even the slightest bit icky, pass on the rest of the dish. It's not worth taking the risk!

Turkey Day Tip #3: It's not called Thanks-GIVING for nothing.

I don't know about you but leftovers bug the hell out of me. I don't like them because I never eat them all. And unlike many of you, my day job involves being in the realities of hungry children (and adults) in Africa. So mentally I can't deal with throwing away a lot of food. To this effect I have a tip and I have some good news.

First the tip. If you are hosting the dinner, give away as much food as you can! Make it easy for people to take food home. I always buy those styrofoam "take out" containers from my local restaurant supply store. They are a godsend. People see those and they think, "yeah...I can take something home..." And then you don't have to worry about it.

If you are attending a family potluck, bring your dishes in aluminum pans from the grocery store — and quietly leave them there! Yes, that kind of sticks your host with all that food but hey, you've given them a yummy treat to enjoy and really? Thanksgiving is a battlefield for us and it's every stomach for itself!

Turkey Day Tip #4: Put down the fork and talk to somebody!

This is the standard issue advice, we know, but it really does ring true. It's not all about food. You will be with family and friends, many of whom will want to compliment you on how great you look! In preparation for the day do the following (and I am serious here, folks). Look in the mirror and practice saying "thank you" in a sincere way. Do it over and over and over. Why? Because most of us only half believe the compliments we get are true. In our minds we haven't lost enough, are losing too slow or just generally aren't doing that great. But it's sort of rude to discount someone's compliment. So practice saying thank you so that it feels natural when you say it many, many times on Thanksgiving.

And if you've kept your surgery private, also practice your "alibi." What should that be? I can't say. I do find, however, that a version of the truth that leaves out that crucial detail works. For example: Aunt Martha says, "You look GREAT! How'd you lose all that weight?" You say, "I've made a lot of changes to how I eat and I'm more active. I'm so flattered you noticed!" See? Simple.

Turkey Day Tip #5: DON'T starve yourself to get to the big event.

That never ends well. Your pouch will be pissy and you'll likely not get to really enjoy your food. Instead, relax. Eat a little, talk a little, laugh a LOT! That's an order!

Holiday Parties

One thing most of us (save for Ebeneezer Scrooge) can count on during the holiday season is being invited to a party. It may be a family party. It may be an office or a church party. But at some point during the months of November and December you are most surely going to be invited to somebody's party!

You all know I'm all for moderation, but once you get to the seventh party, moderation has sort of abandoned you four parties ago! So what do you do? How do you survive without totally back tracking? Here are some tips.

Holiday Party Survival Tip #1: Get Organized!

Sit down with a calendar and mark all the holiday parties to which you've been invited. If you don't have all your invites, also make a list of all parties to which you anticipate being invited. You might also develop a rating system of some sort based on how much you really want to go to that party. Because, in reality, it's okay to say no. It's okay to say that you're really busy and you're so sorry you can't make it and that you hope they have a great holiday just the same. It's okay.

But aside from that, some prioritization is necessary. You might rate parties based on the host's willingness or habit of having healthy offerings. You might place special emphasis on potlucks, to which YOU can bring a weight loss surgery friendly treat.

Holiday Party Survival Tip #2: Decide Accordingly.

Decide in advance which parties you'll attend and which ones you'll skip. You have your own unique prioritization methods, so I'm not going to micromanage your process. It might be that you can't skip the office party but you can skip the neighborhood shindig.

For the ones you decline, be polite but firm in refusing. But do hold steady to your refusal. This step may seem oversimplified, but I cannot tell you how many times I have gotten tripped up by conflicting invitations.

And many times there is more behind an invitation than the invitation. If you sit down, look at it all, think it out, you know what forces are working in your holiday invites and how you'd like to respond to them. That way you aren't caught in any office-political, familial, clique tugs of war that wreak havoc on your emotional well-being.

Holiday Party Survival Tip #3: For parties where healthy offerings are likely

Those are the easy parties. Choose the best of what's offered, use a small plate (and I am not above bringing one of my own), mingle a LOT (if no one person is with you too long, they can't contemplate what you are and are not eating and how much), laugh, sing Christmas carols.

A word of caution, however. Especially for newer folks. Holiday parties tend to involve alcohol. You should always refer to your surgeon's advice about alcohol

My program allows it in moderation. However, with my rearranged guts, one glass of wine would have me dancing on a table with a lampshade over my head. That's not a good look.

If you do choose to do alcohol...TINY SIPS...seriously. Trust me on this one. My very first post-op drink (some wine about a year post-op), I shared with someone. That worked well.

Holiday Party Survival Tip #4: For the parties where healthy offerings are unlikely

See here's the deal. I have this belief. It reads sort of like a scientific hypothesis. In order to avoid a complete meltdown, every bad food choice has to be accompanied by an equally or more yummy good food choice. If this is the case, you'll go for the healthy yummies and won't feel the least bit resentful about what anybody else is eating.

To that effect, be empowered to bring something to the party. Here are some do's and don'ts in that regard:

- DO let the host know you're bringing a dish. If you haven't told them about the surgery, you might say "oh I have this fabulous holiday dish I just love to share. Do you mind if I bring it?" That usually works for me.
- DO prepare something you don't mind going back home with. It might be the best thing ever to you, but it may not be a non-op's cup of tea.
- DON'T tell anyone it is particularly healthy. Just put it on the damn table and walk away! Everyone feels like there should be a "healthy food" disclaimer. You're giving them something that is

GOOD for their bodies. In reality, they should be warning people about the simple carb, sugar and fat-fest THEY are laying out.

- DON'T let your dish be the only dish you try. Remember…moderation is key. Chances are there are some foods you can try besides the one you brought. It kind of looks snooty if you don't at least put something else on your plate! Just saying.

In addition, here is a no-fail one liner that gets me through parties where people don't know about my surgery.

> Host: You don't seem to be eating much…(or some variation)
>
> Me: What…you didn't see that huge helping of X I had on my plate a minute ago? You are really a great cook! Can I get that recipe…?

(The above is nice because you don't technically have to be lying. You could have had what seems, to you, to be a huge helping of said food on your plate. It doesn't mean you ate it. And by complimenting them and asking for the recipe, you get the conversation away from you quickly!)

Holiday Party Survival Tip #5: Dessert!

Yes, yes…I get it. Dessert is the crown jewel of a holiday party. In years past it was a goose or a duck. Now it's some sweet confection that's been decorated to look like who knows what. And you want some, don't you?

I'm not going to tell you not to eat it. You are a grown person and can do whatever you choose. Some points to consider though:

- If you don't know if you dump, this is NOT the time to find out!
- This surgery and lifestyle is about making healthy choices. Having a small portion of something you really want is not an unhealthy choice. So many times we set ourselves up with a "pass/fail" mentality. Eating the cookie, knowing that you told yourself you're only going to have one and really only having one, is not a fail. It's a win. You set a limit for yourself. YOU took control. So if you want to have the cookie, and you don't think it'll make you sick, have the cookie. It won't kill you. If it makes you feel better, go an extra 10 minutes on the treadmill the next day.
- However, if you have dessert, you might want to go lighter on some of your other indulgent choices. This process is about trade-

offs. Perhaps, for your plan, it comes down to either the drool worthy spinach dip or a bite of the yule log.

- If you choose NOT to have any of the offered desserts, I usually defer to my hypothesis above and bring a WLS friendly dessert. Again, I don't share that it's healthy. I sit it down, take my portion and walk away!

Facing the Family for the First Time

For some of you the holidays will be the first major family gathering you'll attend after surgery. And depending on how far out from surgery you are, this may be your family's first look at the "changing you."

Some post-ops choose to tell their entire family about their surgery. Some choose to tell some and keep it private from others. While there is no wrong or right choice, the choice you've made does affect how people perceive you — and how you might behave — at family gatherings. So let's talk about this.

Facing the Family Tip #1: For those who have kept their surgeries private

Your lot is the hardest, frankly, especially if you're a new post-op. You can't eat much (at least not in the eyes of a non-op) and that's going to be noticeable, even if your weight loss isn't quite yet.

I personally don't advocate for lying to your family. You love them and lying to them outright isn't an act of love, no matter how you try to justify it. If you absolutely must do anything, I would advocate more for avoidance, which is hard, but do-able.

A tip on "passing for normal." Firstly, mingle a lot. There's lots of family to see, new babies, older aunts and uncles. The thing about people is they only notice what's in front of them at any given time. When I was newly post-op I used to move around a lot with my plate of food and folks only registered what I ate (which was approximately one bite) when I was with them.

In the end, if you get called out, you can go with the standby that you're watching what you're eating this holiday season and hope your family respects that!

Facing the Family Tip #2: "Why are you getting so thin?"

This question will likely come up (if you are at certain stage post-op) whether you've told about your surgery or not. And here's the kicker: your family, especially older members, always think you're getting too thin.

If you told about your surgery, this is when you'll hear how you can "stop losing weight now before you waste away." If you've not told about your surgery, expect questions about your general health (and maybe some theories that you either have cancer, are on drugs or have, in fact, had weight loss surgery).

In either scenario, what's worked best for me is to say that I've been losing weight under the supervision of a doctor. While I probably look a little small to you, Grandma, I'm actually quite a few pounds from a healthy weight. So I'm going to keep on eating healthy and exercising so that I can be here to love you as long as I can! (See the ingratiation happening there? Yeah, that helps!)

Facing the Family Tip #3: If they don't notice

I hear this from post-ops all the time. They've lost 40, 50, 60, 70 pounds and not a word from their families about it! Don't they notice? Don't they care?

Well, if you've been private about your surgery they may have noticed but aren't sure what's going on and they don't want to offend you by asking. Asking about weight is sort of a landmine, if you think about it. Saying you look great may imply that you didn't before. Or, worse, you could be sick! It's a sensitive situation and many times their silence could be out of respect for your feelings or privacy.

If you've been open about your surgery, there could be several dynamics going on. I know when I was newly post-op I had this nasty habit of wearing clothes that were too big. Which really de-emphasized my weight loss. So not a lot of people said much until I wore clothes that fit! But also, if you have a generally large family, it may be that they aren't making a big deal out of you because of how it makes them feel about themselves. And in all honesty, you have to put yourself in their shoes. It's hard to see someone else be successful when you feel like you are failing.

No matter what the reason, try not to take it personally. And yes, I understand there are some situations where the omission of a compliment is, in fact, malicious, but even then, take the high road. Getting upset affects you the worst. You know what you've accomplished. Be proud of yourself!

Facing the Family Tip #4: Don't be the food police!

I hear from many folks that watching others devour the kinds of foods and the amounts of foods they used to eat sickens them. If this is you, keep it to yourself.

This may sound harsh but you don't have the right to take someone else's food joy away. Whether or not their food joy is misplaced is a matter for the other person to decide. It's not your job to admonish them, correct them or advise them, unless they've asked you to.

So don't police your family's food choices. That never ends well.

Facing the Family Tip #5: Don't let your family food police you!

Families are famous for this if they know you're trying to lose weight.

"Should you be eating that?" they ask in a faux innocent voice. And when you call them out they claim they were trying to "help." It's nerve wracking! But again, take the high road! You'll thank yourself later.

If someone says something to you, you can say something as simple as, "I got this under control, but thanks!" If you want to be a bit more explanatory, you can say "I planned for a little indulgence today so I'm good." Or you can just walk away! That works too.

But do not, I repeat, do not let your family make you feel guilty about your food choices! That's hard, I know. But you know what you can and can't eat and you know what you should and shouldn't eat. And in reality, if you don't know, making a mistake and having to deal with the consequences is a damn good way to learn.

How to tactfully (and truthfully) answer the difficult questions your family will ask

Since the holidays bring together family members who may not see each other often, for some of you, you'll be encountering family for the first time since surgery. This, by itself, can be emotionally challenging. If you have elected to keep your surgery private, it can be even more so!

One of the most difficult parts of getting together with family in this type of environment is having to answer the same questions again and again. You can have the patience of Job but after the tenth time you've been asked a question, you may just want to scream!

With these factors at play, it's good to have some stock answers to common questions. Here are some tactful and honest answers to some of those questions and comments along with some ways to react to common situations that come up. Feel free to tailor them to your personality or situation.

"You've lost a lot of weight! What have you been doing?"

If you want to be open about having had weight loss surgery, of course you can proceed to include that in your answer. However, if you want to keep your surgery private, a good and honest answer would be, "I've been working with my doctor and a nutritionist. I've also been exercising a lot more and eating a lot less. Thanks for noticing!"

"Would one little bite be so bad?"

In my experience, this tends to come from an elder member of your family and it comes from a place of love. Usually someone like your grandma or your aunt knows how much you've always enjoyed a particular dish and want you to know that they won't judge you for having a few bites. But my advice is always the same on this subject. If you don't know if you'll have a negative reaction to a food, a family gathering is not the place where you want to find out! The best thing to do is say something like, "I absolutely love your spice cake, Grandma. And one day I'll probably be able to have a few bites but for right now I'm still adjusting so I think I'd better not."

"You took the easy way out/How come you couldn't lose it on your own?"

These questions can hurt. But remember this is a teachable moment. You might consider saying something like, "I know it might look like surgery makes losing weight easy, but just like any other method of losing weight, you have to change your lifestyle for it to work and that's not easy at all." To the question of why you can't "lose it on your own" I think a semi-humorous answer is in order (I'm a big believer that ridiculousness is best addressed by exposition): "If I'm not losing it on my own I'd love to know who is losing it for me! I'll tell them to go to the gym and resist potato chips!"

You've lost a lot of weight but your family doesn't make mention of it.

This happens to many post-ops. There can be several reasons why. If your family knows about your surgery they may feel awkward asking about your progress. If they don't know about your surgery, asking about weight can be a landmine. Put yourself in their shoes. If you saw someone who has obviously lost a lot of weight, would you automatically be comfortable mentioning it without knowing there's nothing negative going on? And, of course, we cannot discount that there might be some jealousy issues going on. In any of these instances, remember this is your family and you love them (at least, I hope you love them), so try to address this in a way that doesn't fracture your relationship.

In the case of family not knowing about your surgery and not mentioning your weight loss, the best approach is to bring it up yourself in the proverbial "So...how've you been?" portion of the conversation. You can mention you've been working out and trying to eat healthier and have lost a few pounds. This gives the other person the green light to rave about how great you look (because, to be frank, now they know you are not on drugs and don't have cancer!).

In the case of family that does know and isn't mentioning, the same applies. You can mention it as you're saying how you're doing. Just be careful not to go on and on about it. This has nothing to do with your surgery and everything to do with social etiquette. Most people get turned off by people who talk about themselves excessively! By all means, talk about your progress and what's been going on with you but be sure to show equal interest to others in the conversation.

"Are you supposed to be eating that?"

Ah, the food police. When your family knows you're trying to lose weight, and especially when they know you've had weight loss surgery, they will watch you like a hawk. Sometimes this is with the intention of helping to keep you on track but sometimes it's because they want to "catch" you for some reason. Again, this is your family so a reaction that is productive is going to help your relationship more than an emotionally charged reaction.

A good answer might be, "My approach to changing my lifestyle thus far has been 'all things in moderation' so I've accounted for a few holiday treats. But thanks for helping me stay on track." Yes, this may seem overly gracious but it really does tend to get the person off your back.

"So-and-so had that surgery and gained all their weight back."

Firstly, this person is an urban legend, I can almost guarantee it. Knowing that, you must understand that this statement is never really supportive at heart. I'm not sure why family members say this to weight loss surgery patients but the best way to handle it, in my opinion, is to take the high road and say something like, "I'm sorry to hear that. This process certainly isn't easy and I hope not to return to old habits. That's why I'm taking it one day at a time."

"Man, you look great!"

We sometimes have a tendency to take the compliments we get after losing weight as a condemnation of our larger selves. This may or may not be true, but before you fly off the handle and say, "What? I didn't look good before?" consider this. If the compliment was given with a loving intention, you might consider receiving it that way. It's entirely possible that the giver of the compliment wasn't thinking about what you looked like before but was simply captivated by what you look like (and, in part, how you behave) now. As we lose weight, we tend to gain confidence and that can show in how we walk, talk, smile and interact with one another.

In conclusion

This is not an exhaustive list of the comments you'll get. But, in conclusion, I'd like to encourage you to take words at face value. For the purposes of getting through the gathering in one piece, assume that anything your family and friends say is exactly what they mean. Don't read into their words. Also, as I've said several times, choose a reaction that will bring you closer to a healthier relationship with your family, not one that will increase the stress between you. Lastly, if all else fails, know that eventually you get to go home and you won't see these people until next year!

Section 2:
Food!

Food Preparation Post Weight Loss Surgery

I always liken being a new post-op to being a newborn baby. Frankly, our stomachs work similarly!

Just like a baby's stomach, our newly altered stomachs aren't built for foods of certain textures. In general softer, moister foods go down well. Drier, firmer foods tend to give us trouble. Introducing new foods should be done carefully and one at a time. We should try not to eat too fast or, yes, we need to be "burped" from taking in too much air.

So, it goes without saying that food prep is of the utmost importance post-op. In this section we'll go over some of Bariatric Foodie's proven methods for preparing foods in ways that are both delicious and (generally) safe for you.

NOTE: Nothing in this section trumps your good sense. You know what foods make you violently ill. The holidays are not the time to test whether or not any of these methods work with foods that have consistently made you sick in the past!

Perfectly Roasted Chicken or Turkey

Most of you already have your own methods for roasting a chicken or turkey and if those work, go for it! If not, here's some help.

- 1 fresh chicken or turkey
- Salt
- Freshly ground black pepper
- Garlic powder
- 1 large bunch fresh rosemary (thyme or Italian parsley may also be used)
- 2 lemons, quartered
- 2 onions, quartered
- 1 head garlic, halved crosswise
- 4 tbsp. unsalted (1/2 stick) softened butter

Directions:

Pre-heat the oven to 400 degrees F.

Take the giblets and neck out of the bird and wash it inside and out. Remove any excess fat and leftover pinfeathers and pat the outside dry with clean paper towels. Place one of the quartered onions in the bottom of a large roasting pan to serve as a "rack" for the bird. Lay it, breast side up, on top of the onion.

In a small bowl, combine the butter, 1 teaspoon of garlic powder, 1 teaspoon of salt, 1/4 teaspoon of pepper, and stir to blend well. Remove any rings, watches, or bracelets you might be wearing prior to this next step.

Run your index finger gently between the skin and flesh of the breast to loosen the skin covering the breast of the bird on both sides. Working carefully, divide four tablespoons of the butter evenly between the skin and the flesh on the two sides of the breast, spreading it evenly over the breast halves.

Rub the remaining butter evenly over the outside of the bird, and season it well inside and out with salt and pepper. Stuff the cavity with the herbs, lemon, second onion and the garlic. After handling raw poultry, always remember to wash your hands well with hot, soapy water.

Cover the bird loosely with aluminum foil and place in a 400 degree oven for 45 to55 minutes. Remove the foil and set aside to reuse when the bird is done. Baste the bird with the pan drippings, coating the whole top of the bird so the skin will brown and crisp. Return the bird to the oven for another 20 to 30 minutes until the skin is golden brown.

The recommended cooking time for a whole bird at 400 degrees is 22 minutes per pound for chicken or 15 to 20 minutes per pound for turkey.

The "old wives' method" is to take one of the drumsticks by the bony end and jiggle it. If it moves loosely at the joint, it is done. You can also insert an instant-read meat thermometer in the deepest part of the thigh; it should read 160 degrees. The third option is to cut into the leg and thigh joint; the juices should run clear.

Remember, it has retained the heat from the oven, so if it is really close to 160 degrees (like 155), don't cook it any longer. It will continue to cook with the heat retained, which is known as "carryover cooking." Allow it an additional

10 minutes of covered resting time (30 minutes total) and re-check the temperature before you slice it.

If the bird is not done (juices are still bloody or it's less than 155 degrees), re-cover it with foil so the skin doesn't over brown and return it to the oven at 400 degrees for another 10 or 15 minutes, then check it again. When it is done, remove it from the oven, re-cover the bird with foil and let it rest on the counter for 20 minutes before serving. This allows the juices time to redistribute before slicing.

The easiest way to carve poultry is to cut the drumsticks and wings off, then remove the thighs at the joint. Slice the breast right along the bone on each side and remove it as a whole piece from each side, then cut it crossways so everyone can get a piece of breast meat.

The Bariatric Foodie Secret to Marinating Meat

Some of you have smaller gatherings and prefer to serve individual cuts of meat. I learned this meat marinating technique from a friend of mine of Indian descent. Her method is quite common in Indian cooking and it has always yielded moist meat — even on the reheat! I've never tried this with a whole chicken or a large cut of beef, though.

Step One: Can be done up to one day before cooking the meat

Season up your meat well with basic salt and pepper (or Mrs. Dash or whatever basic spice you like). Then combine it in a zip-top bag with Greek yogurt and any desired "special" spices (for instance, if you are doing a Mexican dish you might add cumin and coriander, Indian you might add your ginger and garlic, Chinese you might add soy sauce and pepper flakes, etc.)

Step Two: Do this when it's time to prepare the meat

Remove the meat from the bag with a pair of kitchen tongs and shake it gently to remove the excess yogurt. Add any additional spices you wish, then cook it as you would normally cook it. I promise, the yogurt will cook off.

Step Three: Eat!

That's honestly it folks. Wait, that's not entirely true. If you grill chicken or steak, let it "rest" on the cutting board a few minutes before cutting it. This gives it a chance to reabsorb some of its juices and it remains very tender and moist.

A few notes:

- The longer you marinate, the more tender the meat will become. Once I got sidetracked and marinated some chicken for two nights and I could literally tear it apart like paper.
- Yes, this does add a NEGLIGIBLE amount of additional protein to the chicken.
- I personally don't notice the taste of the yogurt, but you may. It's in there. What can I say? But usually if you season the yogurt, then season the meat, the meat will taste like the seasoning.
- I have NOT tried this method with ground meats but I do know it works on smaller cuts of meat, like stew meat.
- Having said that, this does work well if you are changing the form of the meat AFTER marinating it. For instance, if you cube chicken that has been marinated this way it will remain tender. Heck, if you grind it, it will as well. I just can't vouch for mixing this with already ground meat!

In the end, if you want to incorporate things like steak and chicken breasts back into your eating, this method is worth a try. As always, I am a BIG advocate of the "bite test" (take a bite, chew well, swallow, wait a full three minutes for a reaction, repeat once more. If everything goes ok, proceed slowly).

How to Make Protein Pudding

That seems like a random jump, doesn't it? But pudding is a food that lends itself well to the addition of protein. And it's also the basis for a favorite holiday dessert: the trifle! Use this method to make protein pudding for your next trifle. And then wait until after the family raves about your dessert to tell them what's in it!

Step One:

Combine protein powder and pudding mix in a large mixing bowl. Use a whisk to mix them together thoroughly. You can add about two scoops of protein powder per 1.5 oz. box of pudding. The scoop size doesn't really matter.

Step Two:

Add the amount of milk prescribed on the box of pudding mix. While cow's milk works best in most store-bought puddings, some of my readers have reported success with soy and/or almond milk by using less of it than prescribed on the box. If you do this, you do so at your own risk. My official recommendation is cow's milk! But please note that lactose-free milk works, as does cow's milk with reduced fat. Those are both great options for cutting the calories of your pudding!

Step Three:

Using a hand mixer on medium speed, mix the milk and powder mixture until it is well combined. If it is still a bit lumpy, you can break out an immersion blender. Some people also prefer to go from step one to combining with milk in a big pitcher blender. The choice is yours!

The most important part of this technique is making sure your protein and pudding mix are well combined before introducing it to milk. Think of protein powder like an egg. If you don't incorporate it well as a raw ingredient it'll be obvious in the finished product!

How to Make a Hot Protein Drink

I always include these instructions for my new readers. Sometimes no food is going to work but I've included a few holiday themed hot drinks that can still put you in a festive mood. Here's how you make a smooth, lump-free hot drink.

Step One:

In a large cup or mug, mix together your protein powder and whatever flavor additives you'll use (no-calorie sweetener, cocoa powder, instant decaf coffee, etc.).

Step Two:

Add just enough cold milk (or room temperature water) to form a thick paste (usually an ounce or two) that resembles pudding before it is totally set. Then stir well until it is lump-free. You want to make very sure it is lump-free because any powder not incorporated into this liquid is going to form rubbery balls of protein when combined with the hot liquid.

Step Three:

At this point you can add boiling hot water. (And by the way it is a myth that protein consumed at high temperatures is of no use to the body. Again, think of an egg. When it's raw the protein is in one form. When you cook it, it changes form but it still gives your body protein!). Just be sure to stir as you're adding the hot water and add the water slowly. I usually do it a third at a time, stirring after each addition (sort of like tempering an egg).

It may take a few tries but what you should get is a smooth, lump-free hot drink. If it's not hot enough for you at this point, it's safe to stick in the microwave to get it to where you want it. Feel free to top with whipped cream or any desired accoutrements.

Ok, so let's talk troubleshooting.

"Nik, my hot drink is sludgy and thick!"

Use a bigger cup and add more water to your drink. Or use the same cup and less protein powder. Either way, that should yield a thinner drink.

"Nik, mine still had floaties! Blech!"

This could be for several reasons. You might have had a lump in your protein paste. Or you may have added the water too quickly. Or you may not have stirred enough at some stage. It sometimes takes a few tries to get it right.

"Nik, what's this frothy stuff at the top of my drink?"

Yes, there is that. Surprisingly, it isn't just from the protein. If you use no-calorie sweetener, it froths up when you heat it as well. Give your drink a stir to get the sweetener incorporated. What's left you can either keep (it's a similar consistency as the froth on a latte) or skim it off. Your choice.

"Nik, I got it right! But now I'm addicted to hot protein drinks!"

Ok...and the problem is...?

What you won't find on the pages that follow

There are two distinct things you won't find on the pages that follow that you might be accustomed to finding in other recipe books geared toward weight loss.

Nutrition Information

There is no nutrition information provided for my recipes and that is by design. With any dish, there are a lot of variables that affect the nutritional content. Use of a different brand or kind of ingredient than I use in the recipe can cause some significant differences in caloric content.

However, please know that all Bariatric Foodie recipes are designed to be lower-calorie, lower carb and, if appropriate, higher protein, than their traditional counterparts. There are places where recipes use traditional ingredients like butter or bacon. It's completely up to you to substitute as you feel necessary for a dish to work in your eating plan.

I've given instructions on how to calculate nutritional data within this book and I hope you'll give that section a read!

Pictures

No, there aren't any pictures of the dishes in this book. There's a very simple reason. Printing a book with full color pictures costs a good deal and I'd have to pass that cost onto you! The good news is that many of these dishes appear, with photos, on Bariatric Foodie. I've noted recipes that appear on the blog so that you can search them by name and see what the final product looks like. Many times there are also photos of the various preparation stages of the product.

A Note to Foodies Who Keep Kosher

You'll notice some recipes are labeled "kosher-friendly." This is because the recipes were developed by my dear friend and long-time Foodie Joy Muller, who runs a great food blog called *Kosher Bariatric* (www.kosherbariatric.com). Please check her blog out when you get the time.

I point that out to say that these recipes come from her experience as a post-op who keeps kosher. They are not my imaginings of such dishes! There may be other dishes in this book that are appropriate for kosher cooking, but I've only labeled the recipes Joy developed as such.

How to figure out a recipe's nutritional information

Alas, that includes the information in this book. I don't give nutritional information for my recipes because the ingredients we all use or have access to can vary widely. And I've found there can be a significant difference between certain brands. But here's how you can figure out the nutritional information on any recipe pretty easily.

Online method:

Step One: Get to Tracking!!!

Log into (or join) an online food tracker (like LiveStrong or My Fitness Pal). Most of these sites have functions that allow you to make a custom entry into a daily food journal.

Step Two: Don't leave ANYTHING out.

Log every single ingredient, even if you don't think it has any caloric value. Include no-calorie sweetener and salt as well. Those things are important to your daily intake numbers.

Also be sure to indicate the measurements YOU used. If you tweaked a recipe, don't put the amount of an ingredient called for in the recipe, but the amount you actually used.

Step Three: Divide and conquer.

Some trackers ask you for the amount of servings your recipe yielded. Some do not. If they do, when you are finished inputting your recipe you simply publish it and the tracker will tell you how many calories, carbs, protein, etc. is in that one serving. If not, when you publish, the food tracker will give you the stats for the entire recipe. DO NOT FREAK OUT. It's for the whole batch. You'll need to divide by how many servings you got.

Don't know? Understandable. Some of us pre-portion our foods and therefore know how many servings a recipe yields and some folks cook it and eat it until it's gone. Neither way is wrong. Here are some tips:

- If you made a casserole, try pre-cutting the casserole into the sized pieces you would eat. Yes, the fam might get annoyed at having to take five slices to make a regular portion, but they'll get over it!
- For stews/soups/chili, I immediately transfer to a storage container (even if I am serving it that night). I do so with a cup measure (for me that'd be an 8 oz. cup measure…for you it may be smaller). Do that and count the number of times you ladled out…and there's your number of portions!

The "Hand Method"

For those that don't want to use a food tracker, you can always do this by hand. It requires a little more time and a bit more diligence about adhering to the portion sizes that the particular food product calls for, though.

Step One:

Take down the stats of each food you used in a recipe (from the nutrition label) and the number of servings of each food you used. (That's the easy way. The hard way is using however much of a food product you want and then figuring out the math for how many calories that is based on the serving size they provide…but who wants to do that???)

Step Two:

Add up all the stats from each ingredient. This gives you the stats for the total recipe. Again, do not freak. Don't do it!

Step Three:

Divide that number by the number of servings.

Measurement Conversions

Because Splenda® measures cup-for-cup with sugar, those measurements do not appear below, however here are the measurements for the other popular no-calorie sweeteners.

Stevia

Sugar	Stevia Powdered Extract	Stevia liquid concentrate
1 cup	1 teaspoon	1 teaspoon
1 tablespoon	1/4 teaspoon	6 to 9 drops
1 teaspoon	A pinch to 1/16 teaspoons	2 to 4 drops

Equal

Sugar	Equal® Packet	Equal® for Recipes	Equal® Spoonful
2 teaspoons	1 packet	approx. 1/4 teaspoon	2 teaspoons
1 tablespoon	1 1/2 packets	1/2 teaspoon	1 tablespoon
1/4 cup	6 packets	1 3/4 teaspoons	1/4 cup
1/3 cup	8 packets	2 1/2 teaspoons	1/3 cup
1/2 cup	12 packets	3 1/2 teaspoons	1/2 cup
3/4 cup	18 packets	5 1/2 teaspoons	3/4 cup
1 cup	24 packets	7 1/4 teaspoons	1 cup
1 pound	57 packets	5 Tbsp. + 2 tsp.	2 1/4 cups

Sweet'N Low

Sugar	Sweet'N Low Packets	Sweet'N Low Bulk	Sweet'N Low Liquid
1/4 cup granulated sugar	6 packets	2 teaspoons	1 1/2 teaspoons
1/3 cup granulated sugar	8 packets	2 1/2 teaspoons	2 teaspoons
1/2 cup granulated sugar	12 packets	4 teaspoons	1 tablespoon
1 cup granulated sugar	24 packets	8 teaspoons	2 tablespoons

Recipes

Nik's very-very-very-very-VERY strong suggestion

I'm so glad you invested in this book to help you with ideas for making your holiday dishes better! However, this is still holiday food! **I very *strongly* suggest that if any of my recipes (or your planned takes on my recipes) departs drastically with how you've made something in the past, that you test the recipe before the holidays!** That way you have time to make adjustments to get it the way you like it.

One of the benefits of buying a Bariatric Foodie guide is that I am always available to answer questions! If you're unsure about a recipe or about how your testing turned out, email me at bariatricfoodie@yahoo.com and I'm happy to help troubleshoot!

Sugar-free Whole Cranberry Sauce

It's the condiment so linked to Thanksgiving in the United States that it deserves its own section! Here are two bariatric-friendly recipes.

Ingredients:

- 1/2 cup 100 percent Cranberry juice (NOTE: Don't use cranberry juice cocktail, use the Light or no sugar added)
- No calorie sweetener equivalent to 1 c. sugar (see my conversion guide on page 36)
- 1 pound fresh Cranberries
- 1 (0.3 ounce) box sugar-free orange gelatin

Directions:

Wash the cranberries, remove any stems, and discard any soft or wrinkled berries.

Combine the cranberry juice and Splenda in a 2-quart saucepan over medium-high heat. Bring to a boil and then reduce the heat to medium-low and simmer for 5 minutes.

Add the cranberries and cook for 15 minutes, stirring occasionally, until the cranberries burst and the mixture thickens.

Do not cook for more than 15 minutes as the pectin in the berries will start to break down and the sauce will not set as well. Remove from the heat, whisk in the box of Jell-O, and allow to cool for 5 minutes.

Spot Check: *If you are early out, or don't want any actual berries in your sauce, strain the mixture through a sieve before whisking in the Jell-O.*

Carefully spoon the cranberry sauce into a 3 cup mold. Place in the refrigerator for at least 6 hours and up to overnight.

Remove from the refrigerator, overturn the mold and slide out the sauce. Slice and serve.

Sugar-Free Whole Berry Cranberry Sauce

Ingredients:

- 2 (8-ounce) packages fresh whole cranberries (or frozen if fresh aren't available)
- 1 small orange, zested and juiced**
- No calorie sweetener, equivalent to ½ c. sugar (see my conversion guide on page 36)
- 1 cinnamon stick

Directions:

Rinse cranberries in a colander and pick through them, removing any stems or wilted berries.

Combine all ingredients in a saucepan and simmer over medium heat for about 15 to 20 minutes, until the cranberries burst.

Serve at room temperature or cool and refrigerate. (Remove cinnamon stick before serving.)

Spot Check: *If fruit juice makes you dump, omit the fresh orange juice, increase the sweetener to the equivalent of 3/4 of a cup of sugar, and add either 1-2 tsp of Orange Extract or Davinci sugar-free orange syrup.*

Party Foods

Chicken Bacon Ranch Dip

Search this recipe title on bariatricfoodie.com for pictures!

Ingredients:

- 8 oz. low-fat (Neufchatel) cream cheese
- 1 pkg. dry ranch dip mix
- 8 oz. low-fat unflavored Greek yogurt.
- 4 oz. canned chicken breast meat, drained.
- 1/2 c. real bacon bits
- 1 acorn squash
- 2 tbsp. regular mayonnaise
- (Optional) 1-2 scoops unflavored protein powder

Directions:

Cut a circular hole about three to four inches in diameter in the top of the acorn squash. Scrape out seeds and pulp and allow to sit at room temperature for 24 hours. Once dry on the inside, dip a paper towel in mayonnaise and rub the outside of the squash with it. Go back over with a clean paper towel.

In a bowl, mix cream cheese and Greek yogurt well. Add in ranch mix and mix again. If using protein powder, add at this stage.

Finally, add in chicken breast meat and bacon bits. Mix well again.

Fill the squash with the mixture and refrigerate.

Mock Protein Egg Nog

Ingredients:

- 3 c. skim milk
- 1 box (approx. 3.5 oz.) fat free, sugar-free vanilla instant pudding mix
- ¼ c. Davinci sugar-free eggnog flavored syrup
- Optional: 3 scoops unflavored or vanilla protein powder, cinnamon and nutmeg for garnish

Directions:

Combine all ingredients in a blender and blend thoroughly.

Refrigerate until serving.

Spot Check: *You'll notice many recipes that call for protein powder note the number of scoops, not an actual cup measurement. The recipes in this book are designed to work with a variety of scoop sizes, however, if you need a cup measurement, assume one ounce for every scoop called for in a recipe.*

Roasted Eggplant Parmesan Cheeseball

Ingredients:

- 6 oz. low-fat (Neufchatel) cream cheese
- 2 oz. unflavored Greek yogurt
- 1/2 eggplant, peeled and diced
- 1/2 c. fresh grated Parmesan cheese
- 1 tbsp. dry onion soup mix
- 1/4 tsp. fresh ground black pepper
- 1 c. Italian seasoned bread crumbs

Directions:

Pre-heat oven to 400 degrees. Spray eggplant pieces with canola oil cooking spray and roast about 20 minutes. When done, cool.

In a bowl, combine cream cheese, spices and Greek yogurt. Add eggplant and cheese.

Lay out a large piece of plastic wrap and transfer mixture onto it. Wrap it and form into a ball.

Refrigerate two hours.

Before serving, roll in bread crumbs.

Spot Check: *When you finish mixing your cheeseball ingredients, the mixture should be fairly soft, but not as soft as a dip. If it is, mix in more cream cheese. Once you roll it into a ball and refrigerate for two hours, it should firm up nicely but should still be soft enough not to break a cracker when used for dipping.*

Apple Walnut Caramel Cheeseball

Ingredients:

- 6 oz. low-fat (Neufchatel) cream cheese
- 2 oz. unflavored Greek yogurt
- 2 tbsp. sugar free caramel syrup (Davinci/Torani or regular, like Smuckers)
- 1/3 c. no calorie sweetener
- 1 small apple, peeled, cored and chopped into small pieces.
- 1/2 c. walnut pieces
- 1-2 graham crackers, crushed into crumbs

Directions:

Mix all ingredients (except graham crackers) in a bowl.

Lay out a large piece of plastic wrap and transfer mix onto it.

Wrap and form into a ball.

Refrigerate three hours before serving.

Before serving, roll in crushed graham crackers.

Spot Check: *When you finish mixing your cheeseball ingredients, the mixture should be fairly soft, but not as soft as a dip. If it is, mix in more cream cheese. Once you roll it into a ball and refrigerate for three hours, it should firm up nicely but should still be soft enough not to break a cracker when used for dipping.*

Spicy Chipotle BBQ Cheeseball

Ingredients:

- 6 oz. low-fat (Neufchatel) cream cheese
- 2 oz. low-fat unflavored Greek yogurt.
- 1 tsp. ground chipotle pepper
- 2 tbsp. barbecue sauce of your choice

Directions:

Mix all ingredients together in a bowl.

Lay out a large piece of plastic wrap and transfer mix onto it.

Wrap and form into a ball.

Refrigerate three hours before serving.

Spot Check: *When you finish mixing your cheeseball ingredients, the mixture should be fairly soft, but not as soft as a dip. If it is, mix in more cream cheese. Once you roll it into a ball and refrigerate for three hours, it should firm up nicely but should still be soft enough not to break a cracker when used for dipping.*

Cheesecake Cheeseball

Search this recipe name on bariatricfoodie.com for pictures!

Ingredients:

- 12 oz. low-fat (Neufchatel) cream cheese
- 1/3 c. unflavored Greek yogurt
- 2 scoops unflavored or vanilla protein powder
- 1 c. no-calorie sweetener
- 2 tsp. lemon juice
- 1 c. whole grain Cheerios
- 2 tbsp. no-calorie sweetener
- 3 tbsp. Davinci sugar-free caramel syrup

Directions:

In a bowl, combine cream cheese and yogurt and beat with a hand mixer until just blended

Add protein powder, sweetener and lemon juice and beat again until fully incorporated.

Lay out a large piece of plastic wrap and, using a wooden spoon, scrape cheese mixture onto it.

Wrap it and form it into a ball. Refrigerate two hours.

In a mini-chopper or food processor, combine Cheerios, sweetener and syrup until a moist crumb forms.

Once the ball is firm, lay out coating on a plate and drop the ball onto it. Roll until completely coated.

Transfer to a plate and serve with reduced fat graham cracker pieces or fruit.

Spot Check: *You'll notice many recipes that call for protein powder note the number of scoops, not an actual cup measurement. The recipes in this book are designed to work with a variety of scoop sizes, however, if you need a cup measurement, assume one ounce for every scoop called for in a recipe.*

Pumpkin Cheesecake Cheeseball

Ingredients:

- 8 oz. low-fat (Neufchatel) cream cheese
- 2 oz. pumpkin puree from can (not pumpkin pie filling)
- 1 tsp. lemon juice
- 1/3 c. no calorie sweetener
- 1 tsp. pumpkin pie spice
- 5-6 sugar-free vanilla cookies, crushed into crumbs

Directions:

Mix all ingredients (except crushed cookies) together in a bowl.

Lay out a large piece of plastic wrap and transfer mixture onto it.

Wrap and form into a ball.

Refrigerate three hours before serving.

When ready to serve, roll in crushed cookies before transferring to serving plate.

Spot Check: *When you finish mixing your cheeseball ingredients, the mixture should be fairly soft, but not as soft as a dip. If it is, mix in more cream cheese. Once you roll it into a ball and refrigerate for three hours, it should firm up nicely but should still be soft enough not to break a cracker when used for dipping.*

Coconut Curry Cheeseball

Ingredients:

- 6 oz. low-fat (Neufchatel) cream cheese
- 2 oz. unflavored Greek yogurt
- 1/2 c. golden raisins
- 3 tbsp. sugar-free Davinci Coconut syrup
- 1 tbsp. curry powder
- 1/4 c. no calorie sweetener
- 1/2 c. unsweetened coconut
- 1 additional tbsp. sugar-free coconut syrup
- 2-3 sprays low-cal butter spray
- 2 tbsp. no calorie sweetener

Directions:

Mix cream cheese, Greek yogurt, raisins, 3 tablespoons of syrup, 1/4 c. of sweetener and curry powder together in a mixing bowl until thoroughly combined.

Lay out a large piece of plastic wrap and transfer mixture into it. Form into a ball and refrigerate for at least two hours.

In a bowl, toss coconuts with butter spray, additional coconut syrup and additional sweetener. Transfer to a baking sheet and bake at 350 degrees for 10 minutes or until slightly browned and crispy. Allow to cool.

When ready to serve, roll cheeseball in coconut mixture and transfer to a serving plate.

Spot Check: *When you finish mixing your cheeseball ingredients, the mixture should be fairly soft, but not as soft as a dip. If it is, mix in more cream cheese. Once you roll it into a ball and refrigerate for three hours, it should firm up nicely but should still be soft enough not to break a cracker when used for dipping.*

Curried Cheeseball

Ingredients:

- 8 oz. low-fat (Neufchatel) cream cheese
- 1 c. fat free unflavored Greek yogurt
- 1 tbsp. curry powder
- 2 tbsp. no-calorie sweetener
- 1/4 c. golden raisins
- 1/2 c. walnut pieces

Directions:

In a bowl, combine cream cheese, yogurt, sweetener and curry powder. Mix well.

Fold in raisins and blend thoroughly.

Turn out onto plastic wrap and form into a ball. Refrigerate one hour.

Lay nuts on a plate and roll ball into nuts.

Serve cold.

Spot Check: *When you finish mixing your cheeseball ingredients, the mixture should be fairly soft, but not as soft as a dip. If it is, mix in more cream cheese. Once you roll it into a ball and refrigerate for one hour, it should firm up nicely but should still be soft enough not to break a cracker when used for dipping.*

Moroccan Curried Cheese Log

Search this recipe title at bariatricfoodie.com for pictures!

Ingredients:

- 16 oz. low-fat (Neufchatel) cream cheese, softened
- 1/4 c. Greek yogurt
- Optional: 2 scoops unflavored protein powder
- 1.5 tbsp. curry powder
- 1 tsp. salt
- 1/8 c. dried cherries
- 1/8 c. golden raisins
- 1/8 c. dried apricots, cut into pieces with kitchen shears
- 1 c. chopped walnuts

Directions:

In a bowl, combine cream cheese and yogurt and beat with a hand mixer until just blended.

Add protein powder (if using), salt and curry powder and beat again until fully incorporated.

Stir in the fruit pieces until well mixed.

Wrap in plastic wrap and refrigerate at least two hours. Before serving, roll the log in the nuts.

Buffalo Wing Cheeseball

Search this recipe title on bariatricfoodie.com for pictures!

Ingredients:

- 16 oz. low-fat (Neufchatel) cream cheese, softened
- 1/4 c. Greek yogurt
- 2 stalks celery, diced fine
- 1 can chicken breast meat, drained and shredded fine with a fork
- 1 pkg. bleu cheese crumbles
- 1/2 packet Ranch dip mix
- 2 tsp. hot sauce
- Optional: 2 scoops unflavored protein powder
- 1 c. slivered almonds
- 2 tbsp. Ranch dip mix

Directions:

In a bowl, combine cream cheese and yogurt and beat with a hand mixer until just blended. Add protein powder and dip mix powder and beat again until fully incorporated.

Stir in the chicken, bleu cheese crumbles and celery until well mixed.

Lay out a large piece of waxed paper and, using a wooden spoon or rubber spatula, scrape half of cheese mixture onto it. Roll it into a log (or ball, your choice) and wrap tightly with plastic wrap. Repeat the process with remaining half of the mixture.

Refrigerate at least two hours.

Bariatric Foodie Party Mix

Ingredients:

- 3 c. whole wheat rice cereal (i.e, Wheat Chex)
- 1 c. roasted edamame
- 1/4 c. sesame crisps
- 1/2 c. shelled sunflower seeds
- 1/2 c. natural craisins
- 3 tbsp. olive oil butter spread, melted
- 1 clove garlic, minced
- 1 tbsp. soy sauce
- 1 tbsp. no-calorie sweetener
- 1/8 tsp. cayenne pepper

Directions:

Combine all ingredients in a large bowl and toss to coat.

Bake in a 350 degree oven for 10 to15 minutes, or until mixture is crispy.

Spot Check: *If you're in another room and you begin to smell the yumminess of this mixture, it means it's time to come out of the oven! When you can smell it, it's done!*

Hummus*

Ingredients:

- 4 c. of cooked chickpeas (don't use canned)
- 8 oz. Tahini paste (sesame butter mixed according to package directions)
- 1/2 c. lemon juice
- 2 cloves garlic
- 1/2 tsp. cumin
- 1/2 tsp. salt
- 1/8 tsp. pepper
- 1 tbsp. olive oil
- 2 tsp. paprika (garnish)
- 2 tsp. parsley, chopped (garnish)

Directions:

Blend all ingredients in a blender or food processor (except oil and garnishes). Place in a serving dish and drizzle olive oil on top. Sprinkle with paprika and parsley. Serve with cut up vegetables.

Variation: *You can add about ¼ cup of cooked chickpeas to the blended mixture before drizzling the oil and topping with the garnishes.*

---

* *Kosher-friendly recipe courtesy of Kosher Bariatric, www.kosherbariatric.com.*

Mock Chopped Liver[*]

Ingredients:

- 3 large onions, coarsely chopped
- 3 tbsp. oil
- 1 lb. walnuts
- 6 hard-boiled eggs
- 2 tbsp. mayonnaise
- 1/2 tsp. salt
- 1/8 tsp. pepper

Directions:

Sauté onions in oil until caramelized.

Mix all ingredients together in a food processor until smooth. Chill before serving.

---

*   *Kosher-friendly recipe courtesy of Kosher Bariatric, www.kosherbariatric.com.*

Starchy Sides
Cornbread Craisin Stuffing

Ingredients:

- 1/2 box corn muffin mix
- 1/2 c. low-carb baking mix
- 1/4 c. Canola oil
- 1 egg
- 1 tsp. baking powder
- 1/2 c. milk
- 2 tbsp. no-calorie sweetener, divided
- 1/2 c. chopped walnut pieces
- 1/2 c. craisins
- 1/2 c. no sugar added apple juice
- 1/4 c. chicken broth
- Flat leaf parsley, roughly chopped
- 1/8 tsp. dried sage
- 1/8 tsp. thyme
- 1/2 tsp. cinnamon

Directions:

Two days before you intend to serve the stuffing, start by preheating your oven to 350 degrees.

Mix together corn muffin mix, baking mix and baking powder. Add one tablespoon no-calorie sweetener, oil, eggs and milk and whisk (or beat on low with a hand mixer) until fully incorporated. Mixture will be gritty and thick.

Spray a baking sheet with cooking spray (for best results, use spray made for baking which has a small amount of flour in it) and bake at 350 degrees for 15 to 20 minutes or until a fork inserted in the center comes out clean. Cool and allow cornbread to become slightly stale over the next few days (leave unwrapped in a cool, dry area).

On the day you intend to serve, preheat oven to 350 degrees again.

In a pan, bring apple juice, chicken broth, all spices and remaining no calorie sweetener to a boil.

In a bowl, crumble stale cornbread, then add liquid mixture, craisins and nuts, tossing to coat.

Transfer to a baking dish and bake, uncovered, for 30 minutes.

Apple Walnut Sausage Stuffing

Ingredients:

- 2 lbs. lean ground pork
- 1/2 loaf stale whole wheat bread
- 1/4 tsp. ground sage
- 1/4 tsp. red pepper flakes
- 1/2 tsp. salt
- Ground black pepper, to taste
- 2 Gala apples, peeled, cored and chopped
- 1 c. chopped walnuts
- 2 tbsp. butter
- 4 oz. low sodium chicken broth
- 2 oz. no sugar added apple cider (or apple juice)
- 1 tsp. dried parsley

Directions:

Pre-heat oven to 350 degrees.

In a bowl, combine pork, sage, red pepper, salt and pepper. Then brown in a frying pan. When done, drain and add to a large bowl.

Remove crusts from bread and dice into cubes about 1/4 inch in length. Add to the bowl, along with the apples.

In the same pan you browned the pork, melt butter and add walnut pieces. Cook until walnuts become fragrant (about three minutes). Add to bowl.

In a measuring cup, combine broth and apple cider (or apple juice). Add to bowl and mix all ingredients together by hand.

Transfer mixture to a 9 x 13 casserole dish. Bake for 40 minutes or until top of stuffing is crispy.

Three Cheese Mashed Cauliflower (version one)

Ingredients:

- 1 head cauliflower, cut into florets (or two bags frozen florets)
- 2-4 oz. of three different kinds of shredded cheese (some that work well together are a combination of sharp/mild cheddar, blended shredded cheeses like Italian Blend, Monterey Jack, Asiago, etc.)
- 1 egg, beaten
- 6 oz. container Greek yogurt
- 2 tbsp. light butter spread, melted
- 1/4 c. whole wheat bread crumbs
- 1/2 c. grated Parmesan cheese
- Dashes of onion powder, garlic powder, salt, pepper and paprika.

Directions:

Boil cauliflower florets until tender. Drain and mash.

Mix in cheeses (except Parmesan), yogurt and whatever spices you like, except the paprika (keep the cauliflower in pot when you do this). Stir thoroughly, then mix in the egg.

Transfer mixture over to a 13 inch x 9 inch casserole dish.

In a small bowl, combine bread crumbs, Parmesan cheese and 'butter'.

Spread evenly over cauliflower mixture and top with a dash or two of paprika.

Bake at 350 degrees for about 20 minutes or until top is nicely browned.

Three Cheese Mashed Cauliflower (version two)

Ingredients:

- 2 bags of frozen cauliflower florets or one large head of cauliflower, cut into florets
- 3 tbsp. butter or butter substitute
- 3 tbsp. whole wheat cake flour (or whole wheat pancake mix)
- 2 c. milk
- 2-4 oz. of three different kinds of shredded cheese of your choice
- 1 c. additional shredded cheese of your choice for topping
- Salt, pepper and other spices, to taste

Directions:

Preheat your oven to 350 degrees.

Fill a pot with water and set it to boil. Once it comes to a boil, add cauliflower florets and allow to cook until slightly tender (about 8 minutes). Once florets are cooked, drain them in a colander then use a potato masher to mash them into small bits. Transfer to a large mixing bowl and set aside.

In a pan set over medium heat, melt butter and then stir in flour and mix thoroughly (will resemble putty).

Slowly pour milk into the pan with one hand while using a whisk to incorporate the flour mixture with the other. Allow mixture to come to a simmer. It will begin to froth and thicken.

Add shredded cheese and continue to whisk mixture until the cheese has melted into the milk mixture. At this point the mixture will be gritty. Lower heat to medium-low, add any desired spices and cook the cheese sauce about 10 minutes more, stirring often. Cheese sauce should become less gritty and smoother in appearance.

When cheese sauce is finished, empty it directly into the bowl containing the cauliflower and mix thoroughly. Transfer to a 9 x 13 casserole dish.

Top with additional cheese and bake uncovered for 30 minutes or until cheese on top is melted and browned to your liking.

Garlic Mashed White Beans

Ingredients:

- 1 lb. dry Navy beans
- 15 oz. vegetable broth
- 1 c. water
- 1 large clove garlic
- 1 bay leaf
- 1 small onion, quartered
- 1 tsp. dried parsley flakes
- 1 tsp. dried thyme (or one sprig fresh)
- 2 tbsp. butter (or butter substitute)
- (Optional) 2 scoops unflavored protein powder

Directions:

In a pot, combine broth, water, garlic, bay leaf and onion over medium-low heat and bring to a simmer.

Remove onion, bay leaf and garlic and transfer to a crock pot. Add water and beans and set crockpot on low. Cook beans until extremely tender.

Drain excess liquid from beans and place in a mixing bowl. Add butter and protein powder (if using) and mash with a potato masher or mix with an immersion blender (recommended).

After beans are desired consistency, add in dried herbs and desired spices and mix well.If beans are too thick, add some milk, one tablespoon at a time, until desired thinness is achieved.

If beans are too thin, transfer to a casserole dish and bake on 350 degrees for about 30 minutes and then allow to fully cool. Beans with thicken upon standing.

Transfer to serving bowl and serve alongside your favorite gravy recipe.

Sweet 'n Salty Potato Casserole

Search this recipe title on bariatricfoodie.com for pictures!

Ingredients:

- 2 lbs. sweet potatoes
- 3 scoops unflavored protein powder
- 1 egg, beaten
- 1/2 c. fat-free evaporated milk
- 3/4 c. no-calorie sweetener
- 1 tsp. pumpkin pie spice
- Topping:
  - 3 tbsp. butter
  - 1 tsp. salt
  - 2 c. chopped pecans

Directions:

Pre-heat oven to 400 degrees.

Spray whole sweet potatoes with canola oil non-stick cooking spray and place on a baking sheet. Roast for 30 to40 minutes or until a fork easily pierces the potatoes.

Remove from oven and allow to cool. Lower oven temperature to 350 degrees. Using a clean dish cloth, rub the skins off the sweet potatoes and discard. Add potatoes to a bowl.

Add protein powder, evaporated milk, sweetener and pumpkin pie spice and use a potato masher to mash the potatoes. Add egg and mix thoroughly. Mixture may be chunky. If smooth consistency is desired, use a hand mixer after mashing.

Melt butter in a pan and add pecans, tossing to coat thoroughly. Add generous amount of salt to the mixture (when taste testing, mix should seem slightly over salted).

Add mashed sweet potato mixture to a casserole dish and spread into an even layer. Top with pecans.

Bake at 350 degrees for 40 minutes.

Cool 10 minutes before serving.

Spot Check: *This recipe is so satisfying because it pairs something very sweet and something very salty, so don't worry if your sweet potato mixture seems a bit too sweet and your nut topping too salty. When combined they are great! Of course, feel free to adjust according to your tastes and health needs.*

Corn Pudding

Ingredients:

- 1 can whole kernel corn
- 1 can cream style corn
- 2 eggs
- 1/2 c. nonfat Greek yogurt
- 1/2 c. butter or light butter spread (like "I Can't Believe It's Not Butter!"), melted
- 1/2 pkg. Jiffy corn muffin mix
- 2 tbsp. no-calorie sweetener
- 1/2 c. low-carb baking mix
- 8 slices cooked bacon, crumbled
- 1 1/2 c. + 1/2 c. 2% shredded cheddar cheese
- 1 tsp. garlic powder
- 1 tsp. onion powder

Directions:

Pre-heat oven to 350 degrees. Combine corn, eggs, Greek yogurt, butter, eggs, garlic powder, onion powder, no-calorie sweetener and salt until thoroughly combined.

Fold in the corn muffin mix, baking mix, bacon bits and 1 1/2 cups of cheese. Stir with a rubber spatula until completely mixed together.

Spray a 9 x 9 inch casserole dish and add batter. Bake 45 minutes or until golden brown. Remove from oven and top with remaining cheese and return to oven for five to 10 minutes.

Smashed Turnips 'n Taters

Ingredients:

- 3 large Turnips, peeled and quartered
- 1 large white potato, peeled and quartered
- 4 tbsp. butter or low-fat butter spread
- ½ c. milk
- 2 eggs

Directions:

Boil turnips and potatoes until soft and then drain. Add butter and milk and mash.

Use immersion blender, if necessary, to get a smooth texture. Add whatever spices you like (I added salt and a tablespoon of no-calorie sweetener to cut the bitterness), black pepper, garlic and two eggs. Mix thoroughly.

Spread turnip/potato mixture in the bottom of a baking pan and bake for 30 to45 minutes (until it is brown around the edges and there is no visible moisture on top).

Don't be surprised if this has a slightly bitter taste. That's the turnips. Garlic makes a good accompaniment to the bitter!

Tzimmes^*

Ingredients:

- 1 lb. baby carrots
- 6 sweet potatoes, chopped into large pieces
- 1 1/4 c. Crystal Light orange flavored drink mix (liquid)
- 1/2 c. unsweetened apple sauce
- 1/2 tsp. salt
- 1/2 tsp. cinnamon
- 2 tbsp. olive oil
- No-calorie sweetener, to taste

Directions:

Combine all ingredients and cook in a covered pot over low heat until tender, about 45 minutes.

---

* *Kosher-friendly recipe courtesy of Kosher Bariatric, www.kosherbariatric.com.*

Cracker Kishke[*]

Ingredients:

- 1 package of Wasa or Ryvita whole grain rye crackers
- 2 stalks celery, cut into pieces
- 3 carrots, peeled and cut into pieces
- 1 onion, quartered
- 3 cloves garlic
- 1/2 c. oil
- 1 tsp. paprika
- 1 tsp. salt

Directions:

Pre-heat oven to 375 degrees.

Place all ingredients into a food processor and process until it forms a thick and smooth dough.

Shape into a roll onto a large piece of greased foil. Roll tightly in foil and bake on a baking sheet for 40 minutes. Let cool.

Unroll, slice and serve.

This may also be put into the cholent (Jewish Sabbath stew) wrapped in foil, then unrolled and sliced when cholent is served.

---

*   *Kosher-friendly recipe courtesy of Kosher Bariatric, www.kosherbariatric.com.*

Sweet Potato Kugel[*]

Ingredients:

- 1 c. unsweetened apple sauce
- 3/4 c. soy milk
- 1 tsp. cinnamon
- 3/4 tsp. nutmeg
- 1/2 tsp. salt
- 3 eggs, beaten
- 6 sweet potatoes (4 c. grated, peeled)
- No-calorie sweetner, to taste

Directions:

Pre-heat oven to 350 degrees.

Combine all ingredients except sweet potatoes in a large mixing bowl.

Add the sweet potatoes and mix very well.

Pour into a greased 1 1/2 quart casserole dish.

Bake for 20 minutes.

Stir once and continue baking an additional 40 minutes or until top is browned and the edges pull away from the sides of the casserole dish.

---

*   *Kosher-friendly recipe courtesy of Kosher Bariatric, www.kosherbariatric.com.*

Spaghetti Squash Kugel[*]

Ingredients:

- 2 spaghetti squash
- 4 eggs, beaten
- 1 tsp. cinnamon
- 1/2 tsp. nutmeg
- 3/4 c. no-calorie sweetener (or to taste)
- 1 tsp. salt
- 1 c. crushed pineapple, drained
- 3/4 c. ground walnuts

Directions:

Pre-heat oven to 350°F.

Slice spaghetti squash in half and place on a large baking tray open side facing down. Fill pan with 1/4 inch water. Bake for about 30 minutes until squash is just tender enough that you can pull out the inside with a fork.

Remove squash from oven and let cool. In the meantime, mix eggs, spices, no-calorie sweetener and salt.

Using a fork, pull out the spaghetti squash and mix into egg mixture with a wooden spoon. Mix in pineapple. Top with ground walnuts.

Bake in 9 inch baking pan for 40 minutes.

---

*   *Kosher-friendly recipe courtesy of Kosher Bariatric, www.kosherbariatric.com.*

Veggie Sides

Green Bean Casserole

Ingredients:

- 1 can low fat cream of mushroom soup
- 1/4 c. milk
- 1 tsp. soy sauce
- Ground black pepper
- 4 cans cut green beans
- 1/4 cup Greek yogurt
- 2 c. shredded cheddar cheese
- 1 can stems & pieces mushrooms, drained
- 2/3 c. French fried onions

Directions:

Whisk together the soup, milk, yogurt, soy sauce, black pepper, garlic powder and onion powder until thoroughly combined.

To microwave: Fold in one cup of cheese, beans and mushrooms, then pour mixture into a three quart microwave safe dish. Microwave on high for five minutes, then stir. Heat for an additional minute until cheese is melted. Top with reserved cup of cheese and fried onions and heat on high for two minutes, until cheese melts and onions get crunchy.

To bake: Pre-heat oven to 350 degrees. Bake for 25 minutes or until the bean mixture is hot and bubbling. Stir and then sprinkle remaining cheese and fried onions over the top. Bake five minutes more until cheese is melted and onions are golden brown.

Green Bean Almondine Casserole

Ingredients:

- 2 lb. fresh green beans, ends trimmed and snapped into one inch pieces
- 1 tbsp. extra virgin olive oil
- 1 small onion, coarsely chopped
- 1 clove garlic, minced
- 2 tbsp. low-carb baking mix (or same amount of whole wheat pancake mix)
- 1 c. skim milk
- 1 c. unflavored Greek yogurt
- 1 c. + 1/2 c. sliced almonds
- Salt and pepper, to taste
- (Optional) 1/2 c. fresh sliced mushrooms

Directions:

Pre-heat oven to 350 degrees. Bring a large pot of salted water to a boil.

Add green beans and cook about 15 minutes or until tender. Drain.

Place olive oil in pan and cook diced onions and minced garlic until onions are slightly yellowed and tender. (If using mushrooms, add at this stage). Add butter and melt thoroughly.

Add baking mix and stir until onions are fully coated.

Slowly pour in milk, stirring constantly, and bring to a low boil. Turn off heat and add Greek yogurt, stirring thoroughly. Add salt and pepper to taste.

Get a dry pan hot over medium heat. Add almonds and cook until almonds turn light brown.

Add sauce to green beans and mix thoroughly. Transfer to casserole dish and top with almonds.

Bake at 350 degrees for 30 minutes.

Asian Green Bean Salad

Ingredients:

- 4-6 c. water
- 1 tsp. salt
- 1 tbsp. rice vinegar
- 1 lb. fresh green beans, ends trimmed and snapped into one inch pieces
- 1/2 c. uncooked quinoa
- 15 oz. low-sodium chicken broth
- 1 large glove garlic, whole
- 2 red peppers, stem and seeds removed, halved
- 1 large zucchini, cut in big chunks
- 1 large yellow squash, cut into large chunks
- 1 medium eggplant, cut into large chunks
- 1 large onion, quartered
- 1 tbsp. extra virgin olive oil
- 1/2 c. sesame oil
- 1/2 c. rice vinegar
- 1/4 c. lower sodium soy sauce
- 2 tbsp. no-calorie sweetener
- 1 c. + 1/2 c. unsalted cashews

Directions:

Pre-heat oven to 400 degrees.

Add salt andone tablespoon rice vinegar to a large pot of water and bring to a boil. Add green beans and cook about 10 minutes. Beans should be just slightly underdone.

In a large pot, combine chicken broth and whole garlic clove and bring to a boil. Remove garlic, add quinoa, return to a boil, then reduce heat to medium and cover. Cook about 20 minutes or until quinoa is tender and rings have separated from the grain. Stir frequently.

Coat vegetables in olive oil and place on a baking sheet. Roast for 20 minutes or until slightly caramelized.

Cut vegetables into smaller pieces and add to a large bowl along with cooked quinoa and green beans.

In a separate bowl, mix sesame oil, vinegar, soy sauce and sweetener. Whisk to ensure fully mixed.

Add to veggie/quinoa mixture and toss with wooden spoon to thoroughly coat.

In a dry pan, toast cashews until slightly browned. Mix one cup into mixture and use 1/2 cup for garnish.

If serving hot, return to oven for about 15 more minutes.

If serving cold, cover bowl and refrigerate two hours before serving.

Corn, Tomato & Okra

Ingredients:

- 2 slices pork bacon
- 1 bag frozen corn nibblets
- 1 bag cut okra
- 1 can (12 oz.) low–sodium diced tomatoes
- 1 clove garlic, minced
- 1 tbsp. tomato paste
- 1 tbsp. chili powder
- 2 tsp. onion powder
- (Optional) ¼ tsp. cayenne pepper

Directions:

In a large skillet, fry bacon slices, then set aside on paper towel.

Add corn and okra to rendered bacon fat and cook until tender and warmed throughout.

Add tomatoes, garlic and spices and mix well. Add tomato paste and mix again.

Add spices and simmer on low for 20 minutes. Add crumbled bacon back in before stirring.

Best if made a day or two ahead.

Butternut Squash Soup

Ingredients:

- 3-4 lbs. butternut squash (approx. 2 squash), peeled and seeded
- 3 tbsp. olive oil
- 2-4 c. chicken stock
- 1 tsp. dried thyme
- 1 c. fat free unflavored Greek yogurt
- 3 scoops unflavored protein powder
- 3 tbsp. butter
- Salt
- Pepper
- 2 tsp. Herbs de Provence
- 2 tsp. ground nutmeg

Directions:

Cut the butternut squash into one inch cubes. Place on a sheet pan and toss with olive oil and seasonings. Roast 30 to45 minutes, tossing occasionally.

In a bowl, mash squash, then place in a Dutch oven, add chicken stock and bring to a simmer, stirring often.

Use immersion blender to puree until smooth and add remaining seasonings. Add yogurt and simmer 10 minutes, stirring often.

Add protein powder to individual servings just before eating.

Vegetable Latkes[*]

Ingredients

- 1 c. chopped onion
- 2 cloves garlic, crushed
- 1/4 cup chopped red bell pepper
- 1/4 cup chopped yellow pepper
- 1 1/2 cups grated carrots
- 1/4 cup chopped celery (omit if not tolerated)
- 10 oz. package of frozen spinach, thawed and drained
- 3 tbsp. oil
- 1/8 tsp. pepper
- 3 eggs, beaten
- 3/4 c. almond flour
- 1 1/2 tsp. salt
- Non-stick cooking spray

Directions:

Saute onion, garlic and red and yellow peppers, carrots and celery for 10 minutes add drained spinach and cook another 2 minutes.

Let vegetable mixture cool.

Once cooled, add eggs and sesonings and mix well.

Add almond flour and combine well.

Refrigerate for 15 minutes.

Form mixture into patties and fry in a non stick skillet sprayed with non-stick spray until browned on each side.

---

[*] *Kosher-friendly recipe courtesy of Kosher Bariatric, www.kosherbariatric.com.*

Maple Orange Glazed Carrots[*]

(perfect for Rosh HaShana)

Ingredients:

- 12 medium carrots
- 2 tbsp. oil
- 2 tbsp. Crystal Light orange flavored drink mix (liquid)
- Zest from one small orange, grated
- 1 tsp. salt
- 2 tsp. nutmeg
- ¼ c. sugar-free maple syrup
- No-calorie sweetener, to taste (if needed)

Directions:

Peel the carrots and then slice into 1/4 inch pieces. Place carrots in a covered vegetable steamer over boiling water for 10 minutes until they are tender.

Remove from heat and set aside. Heat the oil in a large saucepan. Add orange Crystal Light, orange zest, steamed carrots, salt, nutmeg, sugar-free maple syrup and sweetener (if desired).

Stir to coat and cook until heated through. Remove from heat and serve immediately.

---

* *Kosher-friendly recipe courtesy of Kosher Bariatric, www.kosherbariatric.com.*

Cauliflower Latkes[*]

Ingredients:

- 4 eggs
- 1 medium onion
- 2 lbs. frozen cauliflower thawed and drained
- 1/4 c. Parmesan cheese (for dairy) or 1/4 cup almond flour (for non-dairy)
- 1/4 tsp. pepper
- 1 tsp. salt
- Non-stick cooking spray

Directions:

Pre-heat oven to 400 degrees.

Place eggs and onion into a food processor fitted with the "S" blade and process until pulverized.

Add the cauliflower, cheese and seasonings and process until very finely chopped. Spray baking sheets with olive oil spray and place in oven until they become very hot.

Remove and spoon your latke mixture onto the hot sheets and quickly return to the oven. Do only a few at a time. Adding too many will drop the temperature of the pan.

When solid, turn over. Bake until golden brown.

---

*   *Kosher-friendly recipe courtesy of Kosher Bariatric, www.kosherbariatric.com.*

Cheese Latkes[*]

Ingredients:

- 4 eggs, beaten
- 1 c. low-fat cottage cheese
- 2 c. part skim ricotta cheese
- 1/3 c. no-calorie sweetener
- 1 c. almond flour
- 1 tbsp. vanilla extract
- Non-stick cooking spray

Directions:

Place all ingredients in a bowl and mix well.

Spray a non-stick pan with the cooking spray.

When pan is hot, add batter by the tablespoon and fry until golden on each side, about two minutes for each side.

Serve with applesauce or sugar-free maple syrup.

---

*   *Kosher-friendly recipe courtesy of Kosher Bariatric, www.kosherbariatric.com.*

Desserts

Pumpkin Pie

Ingredients:

- 1 can pumpkin puree (not pumpkin pie filling)
- 2 c. fat free unflavored Greek yogurt
- No calorie sweetener equivalent to 2 c. sugar (see my conversion guide on page 36)
- 1/4 tsp. salt
- 1 tsp. pumpkin pie spice
- 3/4 c. egg substitute (or three eggs) + one egg white
- 1 prepared pie crust
- Optional: 3 scoops vanilla or unflavored protein powder

Directions:

In a bowl, combine pumpkin, yogurt, egg substitute, sweetener, salt and protein powder. Beat on low with a hand mixer until fully incorporated. If you use protein powder, include it in this stage, also.

Add spices and mix with a wooden spoon or spatula.

Line a pie plate with pie crust and pour in filling. Cover the crust edges with aluminum foil.

Bake in a 350 degree oven for 50 minutes or until center is set. About five minutes before extracting, uncover the pie crust edges and brush them with egg white.

Cool on a wire rack for two hours before slicing. Serve with fat-free whipped cream.

"Amp'd" Sweet Potato Pie

Search this recipe title on bariatricfoodie.com for pictures!

Ingredients:

- 4 large sweet potatoes, peeled
- No calorie sweetener equivalent to 1 + 1/3 c. sugar (see my conversion guide on page 36)
- 3 scoops protein powder
- 1 tsp. pumpkin pie spice
- 1 egg (or ¼ c. Egg Beaters)
- 1 can fat-free evaporated milk

Directions:

Pre-heat oven to 350 degrees.

In a mixing bowl, mash sweet potatoes then add sweetener, pumpkin spice and protein powder and egg. Mix thoroughly.

Add evaporated milk and mix again (for best results, mix with a hand mixer on medium speed).

Pour mixture into prepared pie shell and wrap the crust edges in aluminum foil to protect them from burning.

Bake for 20 minutes, or until pie is almost completely set. Remove aluminum foil from crust edges and bake another 5-7 minutes or until center of pie is set.

Transfer to a cooling rack and cool before serving.

Spot Check: *The will be smooth, shiny and slightly stiff on the surface…no worries! When it cools, it looks, feels and tastes like a traditional pie!*

No-Flour Oatmeal Cookies

Search this recipe title on bariatricfoodie.com for pictures!

Dry ingredients:

- 1 c. quick oats, halved
- 1/8 tsp. salt
- 1/2 tsp. baking soda
- 1/4 tsp. pumpkin pie spice

Wet ingredients:

- 1/2 stick low-calorie baking butter substitute (equivalent of 1/4 c. or 4 tbsp. I used Blue Bonnet Light)
- 1 egg
- No calorie sweetener equivalent to 1 c. sugar (see my conversion guide on page 36)
- 1/2 tsp vanilla

Additions:

- 1/4 c. raisins
- 1/4 c. chopped walnuts

Directions:

Pre-heat your oven to 350 degrees.

Place half your oats in a blender or food processor and blend into a flour.

Place in a bowl and combine with your other 1/2 cup of oats. Add baking soda, salt and spice and blend. Set aside.

Cream together "butter" and sugar substitute. Add egg and mix until thoroughly combined (with Splenda this is going to look more mealy than creamy). Finally, add vanilla and mix well.

Add wet ingredients to dry and mix until dough forms. Add your raisins in (and nuts if you're using them).

Using a spoon (of whatever size you like, but remember, the smaller the spoon, the more cookies you'll yield), scoop out dough and form a ball. Line your balls up on a sprayed cookie sheet, then mash down into a disc with a spoon (like many no-flour cookie recipes, these don't spread on their own).

Bake for about 8 to10 minutes. And here they are!

Yields 12 cookies.

No-Flour Almond Butter Cookies

Search this recipe title on bariatricfoodie.com for pictures!

Ingredients:

- 1 c. almond butter
- No calorie sweetener equivalent to 1 c. sugar (see my conversion guide on page 36)
- 1 egg
- 1/2 tsp. pure vanilla extract
- 1/2 tsp. butter extract
- Optional: Raw almonds for decoration

Directions:

Pre-heat oven to 350 degrees.

Mix all ingredients in a bowl with a hand mixer, making sure egg is fully incorporated. Dough will be loose.

Use a large spoon to roll your dough into a ball. Transfer to a sprayed baking sheet, then mash down your dough ball with a spoon to form a disc.

Bake about eight minutes, then remove from oven. Place an almond on top of each and press into the cookie while still soft (for a bit of extra flavor, try a lightly sweetened almond from a 100 calorie pack or a cocoa almond!).

Allow to cool on a rack before eating. Cookies will be crumbly.

Yields about 12 cookies.

No-Flour Peanut Butter Cookies

Search this recipe title on bariatricfoodie.com for pictures!

Ingredients:

- 1 c. peanut butter
- No calorie sweetener equivalent to 1 c. sugar (see my conversion guide on page 36)
- 1 egg
- 1/2 tsp. pure vanilla extract
- 1/2 tsp. butter extract

Directions:

Pre-heat oven to 350 degrees.

Mix all ingredients in a bowl with a hand mixer, making sure egg is fully incorporated. Dough will be loose.

Use a large spoon to roll your dough into a ball. Transfer to a sprayed baking sheet, then mash down your dough ball with a spoon to form a disc.

Bake about eight minutes, then remove from oven. Allow to cool on a rack before eating. Cookies will be crumbly.

Yields about 12 cookies.

Nik-a-doodles

Search this recipe title on bariatricfoodie.com for pictures!

Wet Ingredients:

- 1 stick reduced calorie butter substitute for baking
- No-calorie sweetener equivalent to 1 c. sugar (see my conversion guide on page 36)
- 1 large egg
- 1 tsp. vanilla extract
- 1/4 c. Davinci sugar-free brown sugar cinnamon syrup (or same amount of sugar-free pancake syrup + a dash of cinnamon)

Dry Ingredients:

- 1 c. low-carb baking mix
- 1/2 tsp. salt
- 1/2 tsp. baking soda
- 1 tsp. cream of tartar (if you've never used it before, it's in the spice aisle)
- 1 tsp. cinnamon

Directions

Pre-heat your oven to 400 degrees. This was the first discovery I made about these cookies. When I baked them at 350 they came out cakey, almost like a muffin top. They need higher heat!

In a bowl, mix together the butter and sugar substitute and syrup.

Spot Check: *When mixing butter with sugar substitutes, it won't "cream" like sugar does. In fact, it looks a bit like popcorn.*

After the butter and sugar substitute are well mixed, add in the egg, mixing well, and finally, the vanilla.

In a separate bowl, sift together your dry ingredients.

Spot Check: *If your batter is chunky, your cookie will look chunky. So sift!*

Drop in spoonfuls onto a sprayed cookie sheet and bake for 10-12 minutes or until cookies are done around the edges.

Spot Check: *Baked goods made with sugar substitutes generally don't brown well.*

Flourless Coconut Macaroons

Search this recipe title on bariatricfoodie.com for pictures!

Ingredients

- 2 c. unsweetened shredded coconut
- 1/8 tsp. salt
- 2 tbsp. low-carb baking mix
- No-calorie sweetener equivalent to ½ c. sugar (see my conversion guide on page 36)
- 1/2 c. sugar-free chocolate chips
- 1/2 c. liquid egg substitute
- Optional: 3-4 tbsp. of your favorite sugar free syrup

Directions

Pre-heat oven to 350 degrees.

Mix all ingredients in a bowl.

Lump in little piles on a sprayed cookie sheet (mixture will be loose).

Bake at 350 degrees for about 12 minutes or until the coconut is nicely browned. Transfer to a cooling rack.

Chocolate Trifle

Search this recipe title on bariatricfoodie.com for pictures!

Ingredients:

- 1 pkg. Pillsbury sugar free Devil's food cake (to make you need 3 eggs, 1/3 cup oil)
- 2 boxes (approx. 3.5 oz., each box) fat-free, sugar-free chocolate instant pudding mix
- 16 oz. nonfat unflavored Greek yogurt
- 2 tubs reduced calorie whipped topping

Optional:

- 1/2 c. sugar free chocolate chips
- 1 c. chopped and toasted pecans or walnuts
- 2 scoops chocolate protein powder

Directions:

Prepare cake mix according to package directions and bake in a 13 inch x 9 inch pan. Cool thoroughly and cut into one inch x one inch cubes.

Combine yogurt, pudding mix, protein powder and one tub of whipped topping. Whisk until thoroughly combined.

To assemble: in a trifle bowl, layer 1/3 chocolate cake cubes, pudding mixture and additional whipped topping. Repeat twice, layering remaining ingredients and ending with whipped cream and nuts. Garnish with sugar-free chocolate chips.

Party-Sized Cheesecake Trifle

Ingredients:

- 12 c. low-fat unflavored Greek yogurt, divided equally into 3 bowls
- 4 scoops unflavored or vanilla protein powder
- 1 c. milk
- 3 boxes (approx. 3.5 oz., each box) sugar-free, fat-free cheesecake instant pudding mix
- 1 tbsp. lemon juice
- No calorie sweetener equivalent to 1/3 c. sugar
- 2-20 oz. cans no sugar added cherry pie filling
- 6 c. lightly sweetened, high fiber cereal, crushed into crumbs

Directions:

Combine milk and protein powder in a blender until smooth. Add to large mixing bowl.

Add yogurt and pudding mix and beat with a mixer on medium speed until fully incorporated

In a trifle bowl, layer one third of pudding mixture, top with one can pie filling and two cups crushed cereal

Repeat. Garnish with whipped cream or more pie filling if desired.

Spot Check: *You'll notice many recipes that call for protein powder note the number of scoops, not an actual cup measurement. The recipes in this book are designed to work with a variety of scoop sizes, however, if you need a cup measurement, assume one ounce for every scoop called for in a recipe.*

Sugar-free Butterscotch Pound Cake

Search this recipe title on bariatricfoodie.com for pictures!

Ingredients:

- 1 box Pillsbury sugar-free yellow cake mix
- 1 box sugar-free butterscotch instant pudding mix
- 4 large eggs
- 1 ¼ c. water
- 1/3 cup canola oil
- ¼ c. Greek yogurt
- Optional for glaze: sugar-free caramel sauce, chopped pecans or walnuts

Directions:

Pre-heat oven to 350 degrees. Generously spray a 12 cup Bundt pan.

Add cake mix, pudding mix, Greek yogurt, eggs, oil and water to the bowl of your stand mixer. Beat on low speed until ingredients are combined and mixture is moistened, then increase speed to high and beat for two minutes.

Pour batter into prepared pan and bake at 350 degrees for 45 to 60 minutes or until a toothpick or cake tester inserted in center comes out clean. Cool for 30 minutes on a wire rack, then invert onto serving plate and cool completely.

Optional Glaze: Melt some sugar-free caramel sauce in the microwave for about 30 seconds or so, then drizzle it over the cake and sprinkle some pecans or walnuts on top of the glaze to make it look festive.

Spot Check: *If you don't have a stand mixer, use a big mixing bowl and your electric hand mixer.*

Pumpkin Turtle Cheesecake Trifle

Search this recipe title on bariatricfoodie.com for pictures!

Ingredients:

- 1 sugar-free butterscotch pound cake
- 2 boxes (approx. 3.5 oz., each box) sugar-free cheesecake flavored instant pudding mix
- 16 oz. Greek yogurt
- 2 (16 oz.) tubs reduced calorie whipped topping (such as Cool Whip)
- 1 can pureed pumpkin (NOT pumpkin pie filling, plain pumpkin)
- 3 tbsp. Davinci sugar-free pumpkin pie syrup
- 3 tbsp. Davinci sugar-free caramel syrup
- 2 tsp. pumpkin pie spice
- ½ c. sugar-free caramel sauce (or ice cream topping)
- 1 c. chopped pecans or walnuts, lightly toasted
- Optional: 3-4 scoops unflavored or vanilla protein powder

Directions:

Prepare the cake according to the recipe. Let it cool thoroughly, then cut the cake into cubes about the size of walnuts. (Note: In a pinch you can use a store-bought sugar-free pound cake.)

Combine pudding mix and protein powder (if using) in a bowl. Then add Greek yogurt, pumpkin pie spice, sugar-free syrups, and one tub of the whipped topping. Whisk together until thoroughly combined.

To assemble: In a trifle bowl, layer one third of the cake cubes, pudding mixture, whipped topping, nuts and a drizzle of the caramel sauce. Repeat, layering the remaining ingredients, ending with whipped cream, nuts and a final drizzle of caramel sauce. Dust with a bit of cinnamon or pumpkin pie spice for presentation.

Serve immediately or cover tightly with plastic wrap and refrigerate until time for dessert. This is usually best if eaten within six to eight hours of assembly.

Spot Check: *You'll notice many recipes that call for protein powder note the number of scoops, not an actual cup measurement. The recipes in this book are designed to work with a variety of scoop sizes, however, if you need a cup measurement, assume one ounce for every scoop called for in a recipe.*

Apple Brown Nik

Search this recipe title on bariatricfoodie.com for pictures!

(Weight-loss surgery friendly "Apple Brown Betty")

Ingredients:

- 5 - 6 Granny Smith Apples peeled, cored, and sliced
- 3 tbsp. butter or low-calorie butter substitute
- 1 c. + 1 tbsp Splenda
- 1 tsp. cinnamon
- 1/4 tsp. nutmeg
- 1/2 c. chopped hazelnuts
- 1/2 c. chopped walnuts
- 1 cup Honey Bunches of Oats cereal
- 1/2 cup Fiber One cereal

Directions:

In a pan, melt "butter." Add apples, cup of Splenda, cinnamon, and nutmeg and sauté until apples are considerably softened. Set aside.

In a dry pan, toast the hazelnuts and walnuts until browned.

In a blender or food processor, combine both types of cereal, remaining Splenda, and nuts until a crumb mixture forms.

Place apples in a casserole dish (I used a 9 x 13). Top with crumb mixture and bake at 350 for about 30 minutes or until apple mixture is bubbling up through openings in the crumb and crumb mixture is brown.

Protein Pumpkin Roll Cake

Search this recipe title on bariatricfoodie.com for pictures!

Wet ingredients:

- No calorie sweetener equivalent to ½ c. sugar (see my conversion guide on page 36)
- 1/2 c. canned pumpkin puree (not pie filling)
- 1/4 c. Brown Sugar Twin (or other brown sugar substitute)
- 3 tbsp. butter or light butter spread for baking
- 2 large eggs
- 1 tsp. vanilla extract

Dry Ingredients:

- 5 scoops vanilla protein powder
- 2.5 tsp. baking powder
- 1/4 tsp. salt

Filling:

- 16 oz. Neufchatel cheese (1/3 less fat cream cheese)
- 1/2 c. no-calorie sweetener
- 4 tbsp. Davinci sugar-free caramel syrup

Directions:

Pre-heat oven to 350 degrees.

Mix together wet ingredients well. Sift in dry ingredients. Mix until blended.

Line a cookie sheet with aluminum foil and spray it with non-stick cooking spray. Spread the mixture evenly across the cookie sheet.

Bake at 350 degrees for 10 minutes. Remove from oven and transfer to a rack to cool for 60 minutes.

Prepare the filling by mixing all ingredients in a bowl and refrigerate until ready to use.

When ready to assemble, transfer cake to a large sheet of plastic wrap by lifting the foil and flipping the cake onto the plastic wrap.

Cover exposed side of cake with filling.

Use plastic wrap to carefully and slowly roll cake into a log.

Transfer to a plate and refrigerate until serving.

Spot Check: *You'll notice many recipes that call for protein powder note the number of scoops, not an actual cup measurement. The recipes in this book are designed to work with a variety of scoop sizes, however, if you need a cup measurement, assume one ounce for every scoop called for in a recipe.*

Passover Banana Almond Muffins*

Ingredients:

- 3 tbsp. olive oil
- 2 extra-large eggs, beaten
- 2 medium ripe bananas, mashed
- 3/4 tsp. baking soda
- 1/4 tsp. salt
- 3 c. almond flour
- 3/4 c. almonds, coarsely chopped
- 3/4 c. walnuts, coarsely chopped

Directions:

Pre-heat oven to 325 degrees. Line 12 muffin cups with paper liners or oil a muffin tin.

Mix oil, eggs and bananas together in a large bowl.

Add baking soda and salt. Stir to combine.

Stir in almond flour, walnuts and almonds. Spoon the batter into muffin cups.

Bake 30 to 45 minutes, until the muffins are firm to the touch and a toothpick inserted into the middle of a muffin comes out clean.

---

* *Kosher-friendly recipe courtesy of Kosher Bariatric, www.kosherbariatric.com.*

Nik's Banana Walnut Protein Pudding

Banana pudding is a classic, but bananas can be problematic after weight-loss surgery. Try this remix that uses walnuts in place of vanilla cookies for an irresistible crunch!

Ingredients:

- 1 (5 oz.) box sugar-free instant banana instant pudding mix
- 3 scoops vanilla protein powder (scoop size and brand do not matter)
- 2 c. milk (cow's milk is best but you can use lactose-free and/or reduced fat)
- 1 c. sugar-free pancake syrup
- ¼ tsp. cinnamon
- ¼ tsp. nutmeg
- 1/8 tsp. ground ginger
- 1/8 tsp. salt
- 2 c. chopped walnuts

Directions:

Mix dry pudding mix and protein powder well in a mixing bowl.

Add milk and use a hand mixer to beat the pudding mixture well.

In a separate bowl, mix syrup with all spices. Mix in walnuts and toss until fully coated.

Pour half of the pudding mixture into an 8 x 8 inch casserole, small trifle bowl or foil dish.

Top with half the walnut mixture. Repeat ending with a layer of walnut mixture on top.

Refrigerate until ready to serve.

Spot Check: *Please note that if you would like to use a large trifle dish, you should double this recipe. You can also make about four beautiful individual servings of these in glass dessert dishes.*

Leftover Remixes

"Thanksgiving" Casserole (Version 1)

Ingredients:

- 1 batch Smashed Turnips 'n Taters (page 61)
- 1 batch Turkey Goulash (page 94)
- 1 batch Cornbread & Craisin Stuffing (page 54)

Directions:

Layer in the following order: turnips 'n taters on the bottom, then turkey goulash, then the cornbread & craisin stuffing.

Bake in a 350 degree oven for 40 minutes.

Serve hot.

Spot Check: *You don't have to use my recipes to make this casserole. Pick any three of your favorite holiday leftovers! The benefit of this dish is two-fold. Firstly, it freezes beautifully in a foil casserole pan for a quick weeknight dinner later on in the winter. Secondly, since you can't eat much volume, the concept of this casserole is to give you all the tastes you want from your holiday plate in one bite!*

"Thanksgiving" Casserole (version 2)

Ingredients:

- 1 batch of Nik's Turkey Pot Pie Filling (page 93)
- 1 batch of Nik's Three Cheese Mashed Cauliflower version one (page 56)
- 1 batch of Nik's Apple Walnut Sausage Stuffing (page 55)

Directions:

Pre-heat oven to 350 degrees.

In a large casserole dish, add Turkey Pot Pie Filling.

Top with Apple Walnut Sausage Stuffing and then Three Cheese Mashed Cauliflower.

Bake for 30 minutes or until cheese on top is melted and slightly browned.

Can be made ahead and refrigerated.

Spot Check: *You don't have to use my recipes to make this casserole. Pick any three of your favorite holiday leftovers! The benefit of this dish is two-fold. Firstly, it freezes beautifully in a foil casserole pan for a quick weeknight dinner later on in the winter. Secondly, since you can't eat much volume, the concept of this casserole is to give you all the tastes you want from your holiday plate in one bite!*

Turkey Pot Pie Filling

Ingredients:

- 1 lb. turkey meat (or a 1 lb. turkey breast tenderloin if not making from leftovers)
- 2 c. chicken broth
- 2 c. water
- 1 bay leaf
- 1 clove garlic, minced
- 1/2 tsp. salt
- 1/2 tsp. fresh ground black pepper
- 1 onion diced
- 2 carrots, diced
- 1 c. frozen peas
- 1/4 c. low-carb baking mix
- 1/2 c. cold water

Directions:

Place turkey broth, two cups of water, bay leaf, spices, onion and carrot in a crockpot and cook on low about four to five hours or until meat is cooked through and tender. Add peas and cook until done.

Transfer turkey to a bowl and shred.

In a cup, combine baking mix with just enough water to make a thick, smooth paste. Use a whisk or a fork to make sure there are no lumps.

Add flour mixture to liquid and veggies and stir thoroughly. If there isn't much liquid left, slowly add another cup of broth after adding flour mixture and stir.

Continue stirring,over low heat in crockpot for five minutes, then turn off crockpot.

Return turkey to mixture and mix well.

Turkey Goulash

Ingredients:

- 2 lb. leftover turkey meat (or 1 pkg. Fit & Active Turkey breast tenderloin rotisserie flavor)
- 1 c. chicken stock
- 1 medium onion, sliced or diced (your choice)
- 1 large carrot in large shreds
- 1 can green beans, drained and rinsed
- 1 can sweet corn, drained and rinsed
- 2 jars Heinz fat free gravy
- Salt and pepper

Directions:

Put turkey breast tenderloin in a crockpot and add chicken stock.

Set to cook on medium-high setting for about five hours or until fork tender.

In a separate pan, sauté onions until caramelized, then add corn and cook until browned.

Add drained turkey meat, carrots and green beans and then combine with gravy and warm through.

Cheesy Mashed Cauliflower Cups

Search this recipe title on bariatricfoodie.com for pictures!

Ingredients:

- 1 head of cauliflower, cut into florets
- 1 clove garlic, minced
- 2 c. low sodium, fat free chicken stock
- 4 tbsp. low fat butter spread
- 1 c. each sharp & mild cheddar cheeses
- 4 slices bacon, cooked and crumbled.
- Salt and pepper to taste
- Paprika
- Flat leaf parsley, finely chopped
- Optional: Whole wheat bread crumbs

Directions:

Bring chicken stock and garlic to a boil. Add cauliflower and cook until cauliflower is softened (about five to seven minutes) and slightly yellow in color.

Drain and place in a bowl. Mash with a potato masher. Add butter spread, bacon and cheese and mix completely.

Spoon mixture into cupcake cups in a cupcake pan. Top with a bit of paprika, parsley and bread crumbs.

Bake in a 350 degree oven for about 30 minutes.

Thanksgiving Pizza

Ingredients:

- 2 Arnold Multigrain Flatbread thins
- 4 tbsp. leftover Jen's Sugar Free Cranberry Sauce
- 2 tbsp. mayonnaise
- 4 oz. leftover roast turkey or chicken breast, cut into small pieces or shredded
- 2 oz. leftover stuffing
- 1 cup shredded Italian six cheese blend

Directions:

Pre-heat oven to 350 degrees. Place the two flatbreads side by side, a couple inches apart, on a non-stick cookie sheet.

In a small bowl, whisk together the cranberry sauce and mayonnaise. Spread half of the mixture evenly over each flatbread.

Sprinkle the turkey meat evenly over the sauce. Then spoon the stuffing into small rounds.

Sprinkle cheese evenly over the top of each pizza.

Bake at 350 degrees for eight to 10 minutes, until heated through and cheese is melted. Let cool slightly, then cut each pizza into six squares for serving

Sweet Potato Pancakes

Ingredients:

- 2 c. mashed sweet potato
- 2 tbsp. low-fat butter spread
- 2 eggs
- 3 scoops unflavored protein powder
- 2 tbsp. low-carb baking mix (or whole wheat pancake mix)
- 1/2 tsp. salt
- 1/4 tsp. cinnamon
- 1/8 tsp. nutmeg

Directions:

Mix sweet potato and butter spread in a bowl until thoroughly combined. Add spices and eggs and stir until well mixed.

Add protein powder and baking mix and combine thoroughly.

Finally, mix in baking mix and mix once more.

Spray a pancake griddle with nonstick cooking spray and set over medium heat until a water drop sizzles on it.

Spoon mixture onto griddle and cook about three minutes on each side or until slightly browned.

Insides of this pancake will remain soft. Top with syrup or use a Greek yogurt-based dip!

Sweet Potato Frittata

Ingredients:

- 6 large eggs
- 1/4 c. Greek yogurt
- 2 c. leftover roasted sweet potatoes
- 1 medium sweet onion (I used Vidalia) chopped into small pieces
- 1 c. fresh mushrooms, sliced
- 1 bunch fresh sage
- 1/2 stick I Can't Believe It's Not Butter
- 1 c. grated Gruyere cheese
- 3/4 c. grated smoked cheddar
- 2 tbsp. extra virgin olive oil
- 1 tbsp. garlic powder
- 1 tbsp. onion powder
- 1 tbsp. Herbs de Provence

Directions:

Pre-heat oven to 400 degrees. In a mixing bowl, combine eggs, milk, yogurt and seasonings (except the fresh sage).

Beat well until thoroughly combined; you don't want lumps of yogurt in your eggs. Mix half of each kind of cheese into the egg mixture and set aside the remaining cheese.

Pre-heat a non-stick oven-safe skillet and add the butter substitute and olive oil.

Let the butter melt, then add the fresh sage leaves and cook them for just a couple minutes. Remove the sage leaves and discard.

Add the onions and cook them until soft, letting them caramelize. Once the onions start to brown, stir in the mushrooms and cover so it can sauté together for a couple minutes until the mushrooms are tender. Stir in the sweet potatoes and let them heat through.

Pour in the egg mixture. Using a rubber spatula, slowly stir the egg mixture and veggies until thoroughly combined. You want the eggs to be about 2/3 done but still in a solid mass (think omelet) and not in pieces like scrambled eggs.

Sprinkle the remaining cheese evenly over the top of the eggs. Remove the skillet from the stove top and place it in the oven for about eight to 10 minutes or until the cheese is thoroughly melted. Let it cool slightly before cutting it into wedges. That gives the eggs extra time to set up so it comes out in one piece.

Makes eight pie-slice sized servings.

Swirly Stuffing Meatloaf

Search this recipe title on bariatricfoodie.com for pictures!

Ingredients:

- 1 lb. 85/15 or 90/10 lean ground turkey
- 1 c. textured vegetable protein.
- 1 small onion, finely diced
- 1 small green pepper, finely diced
- 1 egg, beaten
- ½ c. Italian blend shredded cheese
- 1 tbsp. low-sodium soy sauce
- 2 c. prepared stuffing, whatever kind you have
- 1 c. barbecue sauce, divided
- Salt, pepper, garlic powder

Directions:

Mix ground meat and TVP in a bowl. Cover it and walk away for about five minutes.

Now come back and add your eggs, shredded cheese and soy sauce. Add the onions and peppers and mix well.

Line a cookie sheet with plastic wrap with about 4 inches of overhang on each side of the sheet. Place your meat on the plastic wrap and press it flat until it reaches about ½ inch thickness. Cover "meat sheet" with stuffing mix.

Using the plastic wrap overhang, fold a third of the meat over onto itself. Peel back wrap and roll the meat again until it forms a log.

Transfer the log to a baking pan, seam side down and pinch the sides closed. Brush with barbecue sauce and then cover with aluminum foil. Bake for 40 minutes. Remove from the oven and cover with the remaining barbecue sauce and bake an additional 15 minutes.

Allow to cool 10 minutes before cutting.

Chunkin' Pumpkin Protein Ice Cream

Search this recipe title on bariatricfoodie.com for pictures!

Ingredients:

- 2 scoops vanilla protein powder2 c. skim milk
- 3 tbsp. canned pumpkin (not pumpkin pie filling)
- 5 tbsp. Davinci sugar-free pumpkin pie syrup
- No-calorie sweetener to taste
- 1 slice BF Pumpkin Pie (page 76)

Directions:

Freeze pumpkin pie two hours prior to making.

Combine all ingredients except pie slice in a blender and blend until smooth.

Pour mixture into ice cream maker and allow to churn 15 minutes or until a soft-serve consistency forms.

Cut pie slice into chunks and add to ice cream maker and allow to churn until fully mixed in.

Top with whipped cream and a dusting of cinnamon, if desired.

Holiday Protein Shakes

Christmas Cookie Protein Shake

Ingredients:

- 8 oz. almond milk
- 1 scoop vanilla protein powder
- 1 tbsp. sugar-free, fat-free butterscotch instant pudding mix
- 1 tbsp. Torani sugar-free brown sugar cinnamon syrup
- No-calorie sweetener, to taste

Directions (cold mix):

Combine all ingredients in a blender and blend for one to two minutes.

If desired, add ice and blend an additional minute.

Directions (hot mix):

Combine protein powder and cold milk in a cup and stir until thick paste forms.

Slowly stir in boiling water. This may take a few tries but if you add slowly and stir constantly you'll have a smooth, lump-free drink. Add syrup. If mixture is not hot enough, it is safe to microwave at this point.

Note: *For more great protein drink ideas, check out The Bariatric Foodie Guide to Perfect Protein Shakes, available in hard-copy and Kindle format on Amazon and in Nook and iPad at Smashwords (www.smashwords.com).*

Mocha Cheesecake Protein Shake

Ingredients:

- 8 oz. milk
- 1 scoop chocolate protein powder
- 1 tbsp. unsweetened cocoa powder
- 1 tbsp. sugar-free, fat-free cheesecake instant pudding mix
- 2 tsp. instant decaffeinated coffee
- No-calorie sweetener, to taste

Directions (cold mix):

Combine all ingredients in a blender and blend for one to two minutes.

If desired, add ice and blend an additional minute.

Directions (hot mix):

Combine protein powder and cold milk in a cup and stir until thick paste forms.

Slowly stir in boiling water. This may take a few tries but if you add slowly and stir constantly you'll have a smooth, lump-free drink. Add syrup. If mixture is not hot enough, it is safe to microwave at this point.

Note: *For more great protein drink ideas, check out The Bariatric Foodie Guide to Perfect Protein Shakes, available in hard-copy and Kindle format on Amazon and in Nook and iPad at Smashwords (www.smashwords.com).*

White Chocolate Cheesecake Protein Shake

Ingredients:

- 1 scoop vanilla protein powder
- 1 tbsp. sugar-free cheesecake instant pudding mix
- 8 oz. milk
- 2 tbsp. Davinci sugar-free white chocolate syrup,
- 3 packets no calorie sweetener
- 5 fresh or frozen strawberries, sliced

Directions (cold mix):

Combine all ingredients in a blender and blend for one to two minutes.

If desired, add ice and blend an additional minute.

Directions (hot mix):

Combine protein powder and cold milk in a cup and stir until thick paste forms.

Slowly stir in boiling water. This may take a few tries but if you add slowly and stir constantly you'll have a smooth, lump-free drink. Add syrup. If mixture is not hot enough, it is safe to microwave at this point.

Spot Check: *In the hot version, omit the frozen strawberries.*

Note: *For more great protein drink ideas, check out The Bariatric Foodie Guide to Perfect Protein Shakes, available in hard-copy and Kindle format on Amazon and in Nook and iPad at Smashwords (www.smashwords.com).*

Decaf Mochaccino

Ingredients:

- 8 oz. milk
- 1 scoop chocolate protein powder
- 2 tsp. decaffeinated instant espresso
- No-calorie sweetener, to taste

Directions (cold mix):

Combine all ingredients in a blender and blend for one to two minutes.

If desired, add ice and blend an additional minute.

Directions (hot mix):

Combine protein powder and cold milk in a cup and stir until thick paste forms.

Slowly stir in boiling water. This may take a few tries but if you add slowly and stir constantly you'll have a smooth, lump-free drink. If mixture is not hot enough, it is safe to microwave at this point.

Note: *For more great protein drink ideas, check out The Bariatric Foodie Guide to Perfect Protein Shakes, available in hard-copy and Kindle format on Amazon and in Nook and iPad at Smashwords (www.smashwords.com).*

Mocha Toffee Twist

Ingredients

- 8 oz. milk
- 1 scoop chocolate protein powder
- 1 tbsp. unsweetened cocoa powder
- 1 tsp. good instant decaf coffee
- 1-2 tbsp. Davinci sugar-free English toffee syrup

Directions (cold mix):

Combine all ingredients in a blender and blend for one to two minutes.

If desired, add ice and blend an additional minute.

Directions (hot mix):

Combine protein powder and cold milk in a cup and stir until thick paste forms.

Slowly stir in boiling water. This may take a few tries but if you add slowly and stir constantly you'll have a smooth, lump-free drink. Add syrup. If mixture is not hot enough, it is safe to microwave at this point.

Note: *For more great protein drink ideas, check out The Bariatric Foodie Guide to Perfect Protein Shakes, available in hard-copy and Kindle format on Amazon and in Nook and iPad at Smashwords (www.smashwords.com).*

Pumpkin Bread Protein Shake

Ingredients:

- 8 oz. milk
- 1 scoop vanilla protein powder
- 1/8 tsp. pumpkin pie spice
- 1/8 tsp. butter extract
- 2 tbsp. Davinci sugar-free brown sugar cinnamon syrup
- No-calorie sweetener, to taste

Directions (cold mix):

Combine all ingredients in a blender and blend for one to two minutes.

If desired, add ice and blend an additional minute.

Directions (hot mix):

Combine protein powder and cold milk in a cup and stir until thick paste forms.

Slowly stir in boiling water. This may take a few tries but if you add slowly and stir constantly you'll have a smooth, lump-free drink. Add syrup. If mixture is not hot enough, it is safe to microwave at this point.

Note: *For more great protein drink ideas, check out The Bariatric Foodie Guide to Perfect Protein Shakes, available in hard-copy and Kindle format on Amazon and in Nook and iPad at Smashwords (www.smashwords.com).*

Protein Hot Toddy

Ingredients:

- 1 scoop unflavored protein powder
- 1 envelope sugar-free apple cider mix
- 5 oz. room temperature water
- 5 oz. hot water
- 2 tbsp. sugar-free Davinci butter rum syrup
- No-calorie sweetener, to taste

Directions:

In a cup, combine protein powder and cider mix.

Add room temperature water and stir until a smooth paste forms. There should be no lumps, so stir well!

Add hot water and stir well again.

If drink is not at desired temperature after mixing, you may microwave at this point with no effects on the protein!

Note: *For more great protein drink ideas, check out The Bariatric Foodie Guide to Perfect Protein Shakes, available in hard-copy and Kindle format on Amazon and in Nook and iPad at Smashwords (www.smashwords.com).*

Peppermint Bark

Ingredients:

- 1 c. milk
- 1 scoop vanilla protein powder
- 1 tbsp. unsweetened cocoa powder
- ½ tsp. decaffeinated instant coffee or espresso
- 2 tbsp. sugar-free, no-calorie peppermint flavored syrup

Directions (cold mix):

Combine all ingredients in a blender and blend for one to two minutes.

If desired, add ice and blend an additional minute.

Directions (hot mix):

Combine protein powder and cold milk in a cup and stir until thick paste forms.

Slowly stir in boiling water. This may take a few tries but if you add slowly and stir constantly you'll have a smooth, lump-free drink. Add syrup. If mixture is not hot enough, it is safe to microwave at this point.

Note: *For more great protein drink ideas, check out The Bariatric Foodie Guide to Perfect Protein Shakes, available in hard-copy and Kindle format on Amazon and in Nook and iPad at Smashwords (www.smashwords.com).*

Hazelnut Chai Protein Shake

Ingredients:

- 1 c. milk
- 1 scoop vanilla protein powder
- ¼ tsp. chai spice blend
- 2 tbsp. sugar-free, no-calorie hazelnut flavored syrup
- Optional: Whipped cream, cinnamon for garnish
- For hot mix also use 4 oz. boiling water (see directions)

Directions (cold mix):

Combine all ingredients in a blender and blend for one to two minutes.

If desired, add ice and blend an additional minute.

Directions (hot mix):

Combine protein powder, chai spice and cold milk in a cup and stir until thick paste forms.

Slowly stir in boiling water. This may take a few tries but if you add slowly and stir constantly you'll have a smooth, lump-free drink. Add syrup. If mixture is not hot enough, it is safe to microwave at this point.

Note: *For more great protein drink ideas, check out The Bariatric Foodie Guide to Perfect Protein Shakes, available in hard-copy and Kindle format on Amazon and in Nook and iPad at Smashwords (www.smashwords.com).*

Where to Buy

You'll notice some specialty items, namely sugar-free flavored syrups, in many of my recipes. Here's some guidance on where to get them!

Davinci and Torani Syrups

The best first stop to find the syrups is the company websites:

- Davinci: www.davincigourmet.com
- Torani: www.torani.com

Use the product locator to find where syrups are available near you. Even then stores are likely to only have the most basic flavors like chocolate, vanilla, caramel or hazelnut. There are many more flavors online! Check the above websites to see what flavors interest you then search for them on sites like:

- Amazon: www.amazon.com
- Netrition: www.netrition.com
- Lollicup: www.lollicup.com

Many in the Foodie Nation have also said that World Market carries sugar-free syrups at great prices.

Low-Carb Baking Mix

There are many varieties out there. On the internet you can find a product called Carbquik, which is manufactured by a company called Tova. Carbquick is very low-carb but not particularly high in protein.

For a high protein, low-carb baking mix, try Big Train's Low-Carb pancake and waffle mix. You can check that out on the Big Train website, www.bigtrain.com.

In stores, Bob's Red Mill makes a low-carb baking mix. Bob's Red Mill products tend to be in the supermarket in the organic or "diet" food aisle.

PB2

PB2 is a powdered peanut product that gives the taste and protein of peanut butter for 85% less calories and fat! PB2 is manufactured by Bell Plantation (www.bellplantation.com), where you can also use the store locator to find it in a store near you! If you want to look in your local store, check the same aisle where peanut butter is kept!

Quinoa

This grain is showing up on more grocery store shelves! Check the aisle that contains rice. But if it hasn't arrived to yours just yet, your best bet is a store like Whole Foods or Trader Joe's. In your grocery store, it may be in the organic or "diet" food section.

Also, search the word "quinoa) Bariatric Foodie (www.bariatricfoodie.com) for a tutorial on how to cook quinoa!

Textured Vegetable Protein (TVP)

This is a soy product that can be used as a filler or as a vegetarian ground meat substitute. Bob's Red Mill sells bags of TVP and those would likely be in the organic or "diet" food aisle of your local grocery store. Places like Whole Foods and Trader Joe's may also carry it.

Also, check Bariatric Foodie (www.bariatricfoodie.com) for a tutorial on how to use and prepare TVP!

Recipe Index

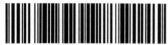

25759057R00071

Made in the USA
Middletown, DE
09 November 2015